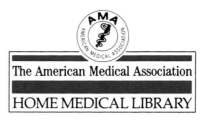

The American Medical Association
HOME MEDICAL LIBRARY

BONES, MUSCLES, AND JOINTS

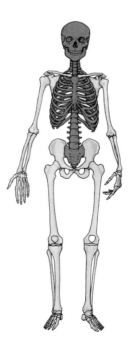

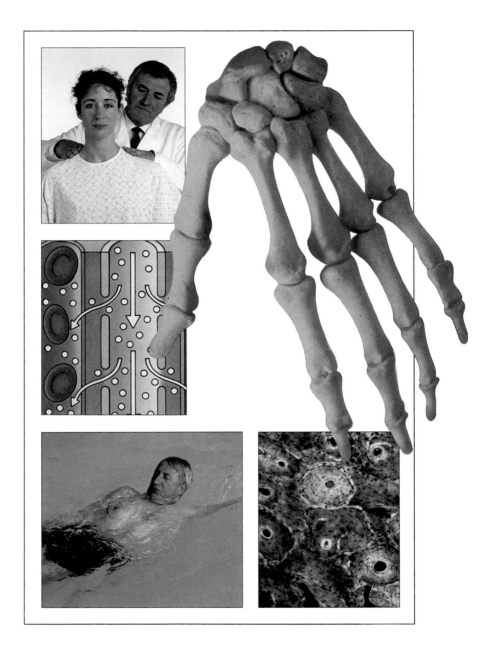

THE AMERICAN
MEDICAL ASSOCIATION

BONES,
MUSCLES, AND
JOINTS

Medical Editor
CHARLES B. CLAYMAN, MD

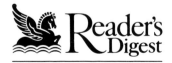

THE READER'S DIGEST ASSOCIATION, INC.
Pleasantville, New York/Montreal

The information in this book reflects current medical knowledge. The
recommendations and information are appropriate in most cases;
however, they are not a substitute for medical diagnosis. For specific
information concerning your personal medical condition, the AMA
suggests that you consult a physician.

The names of organizations, products, or alternative therapies appearing
in this book are given for informational purposes only. Their inclusion
does not imply AMA endorsement, nor does the omission of any
organization, product, or alternative therapy indicate AMA disapproval.

The AMA Home Medical Library is distinct from and unrelated to the
series of health books published by Random House, Inc., in conjunction
with the American Medical Association under the names "The AMA Home
Reference Library" and "The AMA Home Health Library."

Library of Congress Cataloging in Publication Data

Bones, muscles, and joints / medical editor, Charles B. Clayman.
        p. cm. — (The American Medical Association home medical
library)
    At head of title: American Medical Association.
    Includes index.
    ISBN 0-89577-400-3
    1. Musculoskeletal system — Diseases — Popular works.
2. Musculoskeletal system — Popular works. I. Clayman, Charles B.
II. American Medical Association. III. Series.
[DNLM: 1. Bone Diseases — popular works. 2. Joint Diseases —
popular works. 3. Muscular Diseases — popular works.
4. Musculoskeletal System — popular works.   WE 225 B7129]
RC925.B66 1992
616.7 — dc20   91-19163

FOREWORD

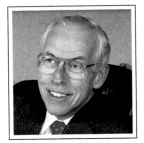

Our bones, muscles, and joints work together to perform many movements of our bodies – from tying a child's shoes to walking to the store. It is important that we take proper care of these structures to maintain their flexibility and the wide range of movements they perform for us. Staying physically active throughout our lives helps keep our bones, muscles, and joints healthy and also makes us less likely to have minor aches and pains.

However, about one in every 10 visits to our doctors is for a musculoskeletal disorder. Back pain affects most of us at some time in our lives, although it usually does not indicate a serious medical problem. The musculoskeletal system is vulnerable to injury of all types. Broken bones and strained muscles are common injuries among young adults. As we get older, osteoarthritis and osteoporosis may develop. Joint diseases such as rheumatoid arthritis and attacks of gout are a significant cause of disability among older people.

Treating the disorders of bones, muscles, and joints has been one of the most successful areas of medicine. Instruments such as the arthroscope allow doctors to better evaluate joint injuries and disease. Techniques now used to treat bone fractures and joint injuries produce high rates of recovery. The ability to replace damaged joints with artificial components is one of the greatest medical achievements of this century. Yet in this branch of medicine – as in all others – the best strategy for good health lies in prevention. Follow a healthy life-style that includes regular exercise and a well-balanced diet. If you begin to experience problems, see your doctor. With early recognition of disease, treatment is most likely to be effective. Many musculoskeletal disorders can be successfully treated and you can return to a vital, independent life-style.

We at the American Medical Association wish you and the members of your family an active, healthy future.

James S. Todd MD

JAMES S. TODD, MD
Executive Vice President
American Medical Association

CONTENTS

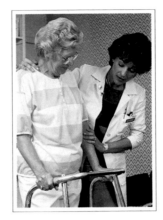

CHAPTER ONE

A HEALTHY FRAMEWORK

INTRODUCTION

YOUR BONES
AND SKELETON

YOUR MUSCLES

YOUR JOINTS

BODY MECHANICS
AND MOVEMENT

Your body's bones, muscles, and joints form a structural framework that is strong enough to support your weight and yet is light enough to allow you to walk, run, and jump. Your bones, muscles, and joints all work together to perform the movements of your body. Our first scientific knowledge of the musculoskeletal system was provided by the Greek physician Galen (129-199 AD).

Because of the difficulty of obtaining human cadavers for dissection, Galen's studies of anatomy were based largely on the dissection of apes and other animals. Galen advanced anatomical knowledge but he also came to some inaccurate conclusions. For example, he believed that, as stated in the Bible, men had one less rib than women. Galen's observations remained the primary source of anatomical knowledge for more than 1,000 years. In the 10th century, physicians in Asia provided more accurate detail of the anatomy of the human body, but physicians in Europe did not obtain this knowledge until the early 16th century. The Italian artist Leonardo da Vinci (1452-1519) made thousands of drawings in which he not only detailed the anatomy of bones and muscles but also analyzed the actions of muscles. Unfortunately, these remarkable drawings by da Vinci remained undiscovered for two centuries.

Our present-day understanding of anatomy really began with the Flemish physician Andreas Vesalius (1514-1564), who published seven major books on anatomy. Although Vesalius mapped the structure of the human body, the discovery of how bone functions as living tissue was not made until the invention of the microscope and the development of techniques of chemical analysis. Such techniques revealed that bones are the body's main storage sites for calcium, phosphorus, and various other minerals. The body maintains a balance of these minerals in bone and in the blood. If the levels of minerals in the blood decrease, the minerals move out of the bones into the blood. Your bones also contain bone marrow, in which most blood cells are produced.

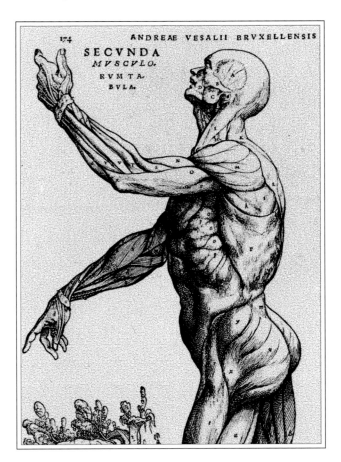

Each of us has more than 200 bones, which differ in shape and size according to their function. The more than 600 muscles in your body are of various shapes and sizes – ranging from the tiny muscles of the eyes, capable of very quick movements, to large muscles such as the quadriceps muscle in the upper part of the leg, capable of powerful contraction. Joints differ in structure and range of motion.

YOUR BONES AND SKELETON

Examining a skeleton in a museum gives us an idea of the supportive and protective functions of bones. However, it tells us nothing about the constant activity of the cells that break down and re-form bone and the interchange of chemical substances that takes place within the bones. In spite of their strength and apparent rigidity, bones are living structures, full of living cells that are continuously engaged in biochemical activity.

STRUCTURE AND FUNCTION

The human skeleton provides support for the body, protects the body's internal organs, and performs movement by working with the muscular system (see page 24). The bones are also responsible for storing and releasing vital minerals and for forming blood cells.

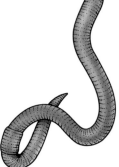

The hydrostatic skeleton
Soft-bodied invertebrates, such as the earthworm (shown above), do not have a hard skeleton. Instead, their shape is maintained by fluid that is kept under pressure by the contraction of muscles in the body wall.

VERTEBRATE AND INVERTEBRATE SKELETONS

Animal skeletons have evolved from those without a backbone (invertebrate) to those with a backbone (vertebrate).

The exoskeleton
Insects and crustaceans, such as the crab shown at right, have a hard structure on the outside of the body that functions as an external skeleton. This type of skeleton, known as an exoskeleton, protects and supports the body and its internal structures. However, an exoskeleton cannot expand as the animal grows. Animals with exoskeletons increase their size by periodically shedding and re-forming their outermost layers.

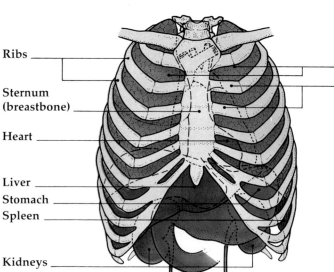

Ribs —
Sternum (breastbone) —
Heart —
Liver —
Stomach —
Spleen —
Kidneys —

— Lungs
— Cartilage

The endoskeleton
Like all vertebrates, humans have a bony internal skeleton, known as an endoskeleton. This type of skeleton provides a strong yet flexible framework for the body while protecting soft internal structures. For example, the bones of the rib cage support the chest wall much like beams holding up a ceiling; they also form a protective shield for the organs that lie within them. The ribs are attached to the sternum (breastbone) with cartilage, making the rib cage flexible enough to move as the lungs expand.

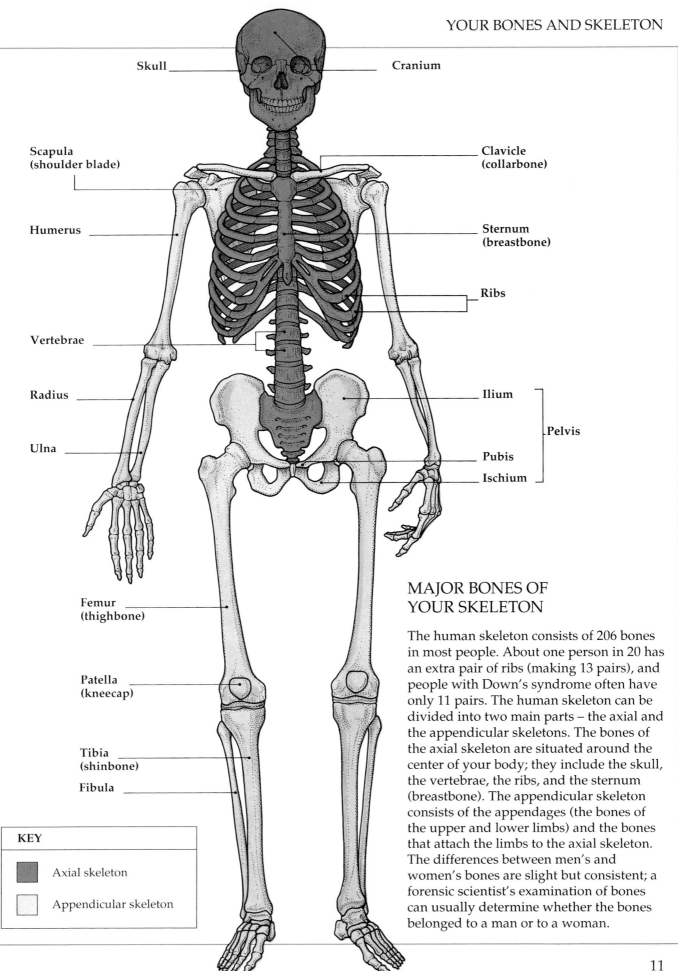

Skull

Cranium

Scapula
(shoulder blade)

Clavicle
(collarbone)

Humerus

Sternum
(breastbone)

Ribs

Vertebrae

Radius

Ilium

Ulna

Pubis

Ischium

Pelvis

Femur
(thighbone)

Patella
(kneecap)

Tibia
(shinbone)

Fibula

MAJOR BONES OF YOUR SKELETON

The human skeleton consists of 206 bones in most people. About one person in 20 has an extra pair of ribs (making 13 pairs), and people with Down's syndrome often have only 11 pairs. The human skeleton can be divided into two main parts – the axial and the appendicular skeletons. The bones of the axial skeleton are situated around the center of your body; they include the skull, the vertebrae, the ribs, and the sternum (breastbone). The appendicular skeleton consists of the appendages (the bones of the upper and lower limbs) and the bones that attach the limbs to the axial skeleton. The differences between men's and women's bones are slight but consistent; a forensic scientist's examination of bones can usually determine whether the bones belonged to a man or to a woman.

KEY

Axial skeleton

Appendicular skeleton

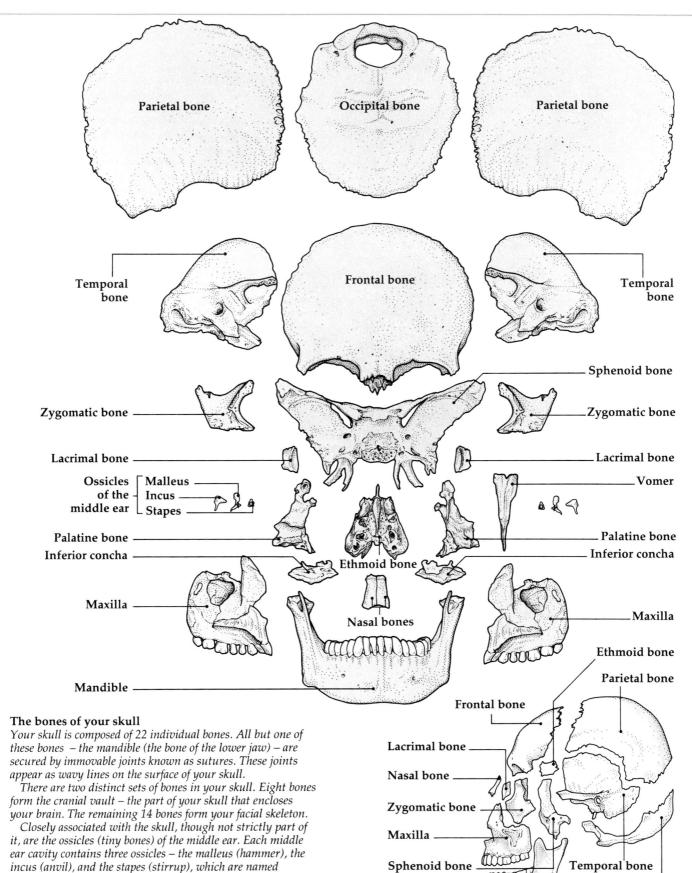

Parietal bone

Occipital bone

Parietal bone

Temporal bone

Frontal bone

Temporal bone

Sphenoid bone

Zygomatic bone

Zygomatic bone

Lacrimal bone

Lacrimal bone

Ossicles of the middle ear — Malleus, Incus, Stapes

Vomer

Palatine bone

Palatine bone

Inferior concha

Inferior concha

Ethmoid bone

Maxilla

Maxilla

Nasal bones

Mandible

Ethmoid bone

Parietal bone

Frontal bone

Lacrimal bone

Nasal bone

Zygomatic bone

Maxilla

Sphenoid bone

Temporal bone

Mandible

Occipital bone

The bones of your skull

Your skull is composed of 22 individual bones. All but one of these bones – the mandible (the bone of the lower jaw) – are secured by immovable joints known as sutures. These joints appear as wavy lines on the surface of your skull.

There are two distinct sets of bones in your skull. Eight bones form the cranial vault – the part of your skull that encloses your brain. The remaining 14 bones form your facial skeleton.

Closely associated with the skull, though not strictly part of it, are the ossicles (tiny bones) of the middle ear. Each middle ear cavity contains three ossicles – the malleus (hammer), the incus (anvil), and the stapes (stirrup), which are named according to their shapes. The ossicles in the middle ear conduct sound waves from your eardrum to your inner ear.

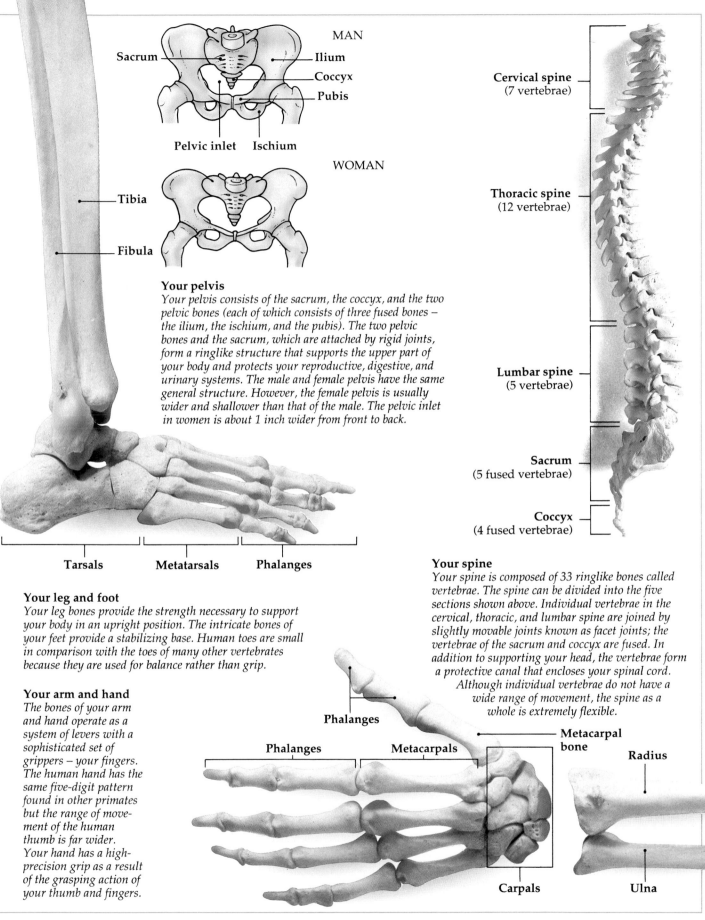

MAN

Sacrum — — Ilium

— Coccyx

— Pubis

Pelvic inlet   Ischium

WOMAN

Tibia

Fibula

Cervical spine
(7 vertebrae)

Thoracic spine
(12 vertebrae)

Lumbar spine
(5 vertebrae)

Sacrum
(5 fused vertebrae)

Coccyx
(4 fused vertebrae)

Your pelvis
Your pelvis consists of the sacrum, the coccyx, and the two pelvic bones (each of which consists of three fused bones – the ilium, the ischium, and the pubis). The two pelvic bones and the sacrum, which are attached by rigid joints, form a ringlike structure that supports the upper part of your body and protects your reproductive, digestive, and urinary systems. The male and female pelvis have the same general structure. However, the female pelvis is usually wider and shallower than that of the male. The pelvic inlet in women is about 1 inch wider from front to back.

Tarsals   Metatarsals   Phalanges

Your leg and foot
Your leg bones provide the strength necessary to support your body in an upright position. The intricate bones of your feet provide a stabilizing base. Human toes are small in comparison with the toes of many other vertebrates because they are used for balance rather than grip.

Your spine
Your spine is composed of 33 ringlike bones called vertebrae. The spine can be divided into the five sections shown above. Individual vertebrae in the cervical, thoracic, and lumbar spine are joined by slightly movable joints known as facet joints; the vertebrae of the sacrum and coccyx are fused. In addition to supporting your head, the vertebrae form a protective canal that encloses your spinal cord. Although individual vertebrae do not have a wide range of movement, the spine as a whole is extremely flexible.

Your arm and hand
The bones of your arm and hand operate as a system of levers with a sophisticated set of grippers – your fingers. The human hand has the same five-digit pattern found in other primates but the range of movement of the human thumb is far wider. Your hand has a high-precision grip as a result of the grasping action of your thumb and fingers.

Phalanges

Phalanges   Metacarpals

Metacarpal
bone

Radius

Carpals

Ulna

THE STRUCTURE OF MATURE BONE

There are two types of mature bone tissue – cortical (hard) bone and cancellous (spongy) bone. Developing bones are initially formed of cartilage (see page 23) and spongy bone. As bones mature, cartilage becomes calcified and the spongy bone is surrounded by a layer of hard bone. The bones of the skeleton vary in shape but share certain characteristics. Some of the features of a typical bone are shown in this illustration of the femur.

Periosteum
The periosteum is a thin membrane that covers all bone surfaces except those at the ends of bones. The periosteum contains nerves and blood vessels and is essential to the growth and formation of new bone.

Medullary canal

Vein

Artery

Haversian system (osteon)

Hard bone

Spongy bone

Diaphysis (shaft)

Bone marrow
Bone marrow is stored in the cavities of spongy bone and in the medullary (central) canal of long bones. There are two types of marrow – red marrow, in which blood cells are formed, and yellow marrow, which is mainly fat. At birth, all bones contain red marrow. However, red marrow is gradually replaced in most bones by yellow marrow. Red marrow remains near the ends of long bones close to the joints and in the vertebrae, breastbone, ribs, collarbones, shoulder blades, pelvis, and skull bones.

WHAT ARE BONES MADE OF?

Bone is a living, constantly changing connective tissue (the material that binds together and supports various structures in the body). Like other connective tissues of the body, bone consists of different types of cells and a framework made of the structural protein called collagen. What makes bone different from other connective tissues is that the soft components of bone contain dense deposits of calcium salts. This deposition of calcium salts, known as calcification, gives bone its strength and accounts for more than 60 percent of its weight.

Because bones are partly composed of minerals (such as calcium and phosphorus), they are able to function as a storage pool for these minerals. When the levels

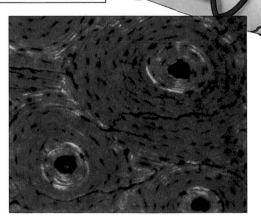

Hard bone
The color-enhanced photograph at left shows the structure of hard bone in cross section (magnified 75 times). The circular structures, called haversian systems or osteons, are composed of concentrically arranged layers of collagen, which enclose a tiny, central canal – the haversian canal. The canals, visible here in black, contain blood vessels and nerve cells. Spaces (small black dots) between the collagen layers contain osteocytes, the cells responsible for maintaining bone tissues.

REABSORPTION AND REMODELING OF BONE

A tree grows by adding to previous growth; it is made up of wood from all stages of its life. However, as bones develop into their mature shape, they are continually rebuilt, a process called remodeling. Parts of the bone are broken down (reabsorbed) and built up again. The process of remodeling helps maintain the shape and proportion of bones while they grow and restores bone to its original shape after a fracture. Remodeling of bone continues throughout life. The breakdown of bone tissue is carried out by bone cells called osteoclasts, which secrete enzymes to break down collagen and release calcium salts for use by the body. Bone cells known as osteoblasts form new bone. Osteoblasts cause the calcium salts to be deposited on the cartilage that will form the bone.

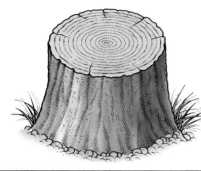

The age of a tree
You can tell a tree's age by counting the number of rings inside its trunk. Each ring represents a year's growth.

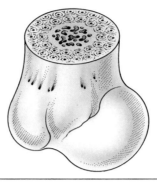

The age of a bone
Bone tissue is continuously being replaced, so the inside of a bone does not show its stages of growth. To help establish the age of a bone, closure of the joints in the skull and certain external features (such as wear) are studied.

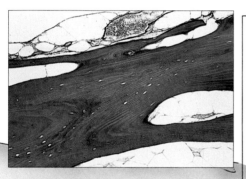

Spongy bone
The color-enhanced photograph above shows a cross section of spongy bone (magnified 62 times). This type of bone is composed of a network of hardened tissues (colored brown here). These tissues act as stress-bearing beams and so they are called trabeculae, which means "little beams." The white areas in the picture are bone marrow, which is stored in the cavities between trabeculae.

Epiphyses
Bone growth takes place at the epiphyses, located near the ends of bones. The epiphyses are composed largely of spongy bone, covered by a thin layer of hard bone. Until puberty, they are joined to the diaphysis (shaft of a bone) by a layer of cartilage (the epiphyseal plate) that ossifies, or hardens, when bone growth is completed. A fracture at the growing end may disrupt growth, causing the bone to be shorter than normal.

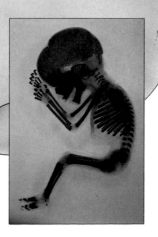

The fetal skeleton
This color-enhanced X-ray shows bone development in a 16-week-old fetus (shown at ¼ its actual size). Skeletal tissues that have developed into bone are stained purple; areas of tissue that consist of cartilage remain white. The breastbone, the carpal bones of the hands, the tarsal bones of the feet, the ends of the long bones, and small areas of the skull have not yet ossified (hardened).

of these minerals in the blood drop, they are released from bone tissue to maintain the delicate balance in the blood.

BONE FORMATION AND GROWTH

The formation of bone tissue is called ossification. Most bones develop from continuously growing bone-shaped pieces of cartilage that are gradually ossified (hardened) to become bone. Some bones, such as the flat skull bones and the clavicles (collarbones), form in membranes that develop in the skin of the embryo. These membranes are condensed areas of connective tissue that become the outer, bone-forming membrane (periosteum) of the bone.

Factors affecting growth

Bone growth is stimulated by thyroid, growth, and sex hormones. Growth hormone acts indirectly on the epiphyseal (growth) plates of bones; the activity of growth hormone determines how tall you will become. Insufficient intake of calcium or vitamins A, C, or D also inhibits the development of healthy bones.

YOUR MUSCLES

Movement of the human body is generated by the contraction (shortening) of one set of skeletal muscles and the relaxation (lengthening) of an opposing set of muscles. The muscles act on the bones to which they are attached. The force that is created by muscle contraction causes movement of bones at their joints (see page 26).

Each muscle is made up of thousands of long, thin, cylindrical muscle cells called muscle fibers. The structure of the muscle fibers is highly specialized and enables the muscle fibers to shorten when stimulated by signals from the body's nervous system. Shortening of the fibers is what causes a muscle to contract.

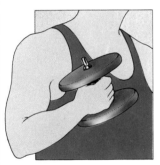

Muscles of the upper arm
These muscles work together to flex and extend your forearm at the elbow.

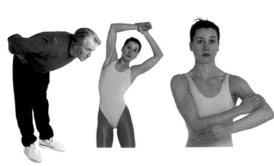

Muscles of the abdomen
These muscles tighten the abdominal wall when you lift or push and they protect your abdominal organs. The layers of muscles running up and down, across, and diagonally in the abdomen allow the trunk of your body to move forward or sideways or to twist.

Greater zygomatic muscle
This long, narrow muscle produces the facial movements that occur when you laugh and smile.

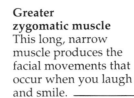

Greater pectoral muscle
This large, triangular-shaped muscle pulls your arm forward and upward and in and toward your chest and side.

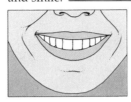

Great adductor muscle
This triangular-shaped muscle draws your leg inward (as when you are riding a horse).

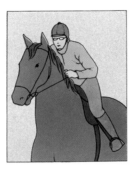

Orbicular muscle of the eye
This circular muscle closes the eyelids and wrinkles the forehead.

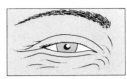

FRONT VIEW

Sternocleidomastoid muscle
This long, narrow neck muscle tilts and turns your head.

Biceps muscle of arm

Triceps muscle of arm

Brachial muscle

External oblique abdominal muscle

Internal oblique abdominal muscle

Brachioradial muscle

Radial flexor muscle of wrist

Ulnar flexor muscle of wrist

Transverse abdominal muscle

Rectus abdominal muscle

Sartorius muscle

Quadriceps muscle
This powerful muscle (long and spindle shaped) straightens your leg at the knee when you run or jump.

Anterior tibial muscle
This spindle-shaped muscle of the shin flexes your foot and supports the arch of your foot as you walk and run.

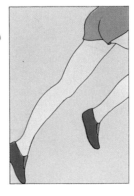

BACK VIEW

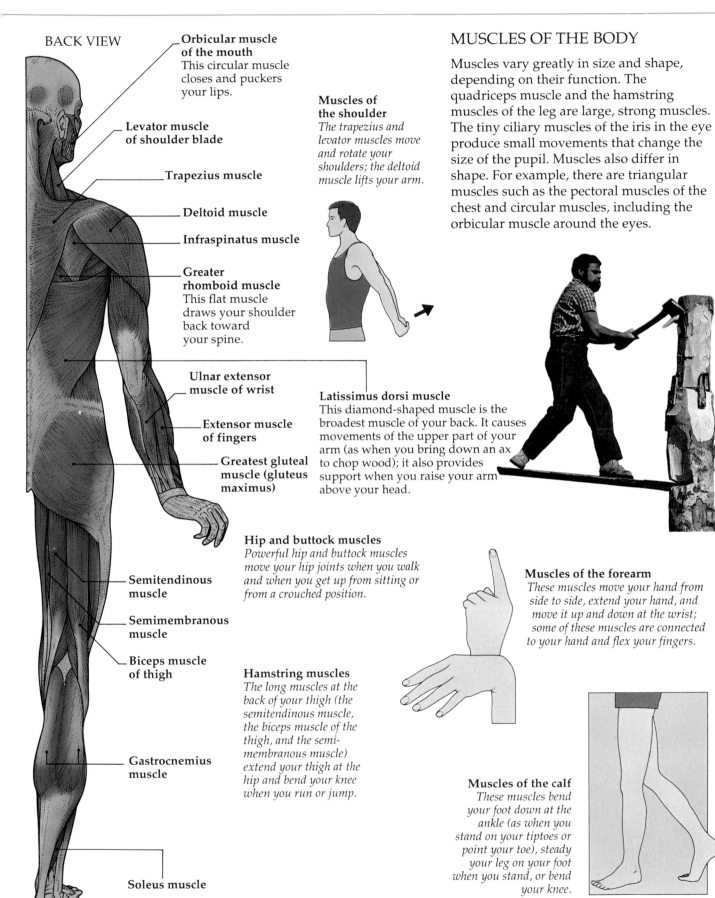

Orbicular muscle of the mouth
This circular muscle closes and puckers your lips.

Levator muscle of shoulder blade

Trapezius muscle

Deltoid muscle

Infraspinatus muscle

Greater rhomboid muscle
This flat muscle draws your shoulder back toward your spine.

Ulnar extensor muscle of wrist

Extensor muscle of fingers

Greatest gluteal muscle (gluteus maximus)

Semitendinous muscle

Semimembranous muscle

Biceps muscle of thigh

Gastrocnemius muscle

Soleus muscle

Muscles of the shoulder
The trapezius and levator muscles move and rotate your shoulders; the deltoid muscle lifts your arm.

Latissimus dorsi muscle
This diamond-shaped muscle is the broadest muscle of your back. It causes movements of the upper part of your arm (as when you bring down an ax to chop wood); it also provides support when you raise your arm above your head.

Hip and buttock muscles
Powerful hip and buttock muscles move your hip joints when you walk and when you get up from sitting or from a crouched position.

Hamstring muscles
The long muscles at the back of your thigh (the semitendinous muscle, the biceps muscle of the thigh, and the semi-membranous muscle) extend your thigh at the hip and bend your knee when you run or jump.

Muscles of the forearm
These muscles move your hand from side to side, extend your hand, and move it up and down at the wrist; some of these muscles are connected to your hand and flex your fingers.

Muscles of the calf
These muscles bend your foot down at the ankle (as when you stand on your tiptoes or point your toe), steady your leg on your foot when you stand, or bend your knee.

MUSCLES OF THE BODY

Muscles vary greatly in size and shape, depending on their function. The quadriceps muscle and the hamstring muscles of the leg are large, strong muscles. The tiny ciliary muscles of the iris in the eye produce small movements that change the size of the pupil. Muscles also differ in shape. For example, there are triangular muscles such as the pectoral muscles of the chest and circular muscles, including the orbicular muscle around the eyes.

WHAT ARE MUSCLES MADE OF?

Despite variations in shape and size, all muscles have essentially the same structure. The structure of your muscles enables them to contract. Contraction of your skeletal muscles allows you to move.

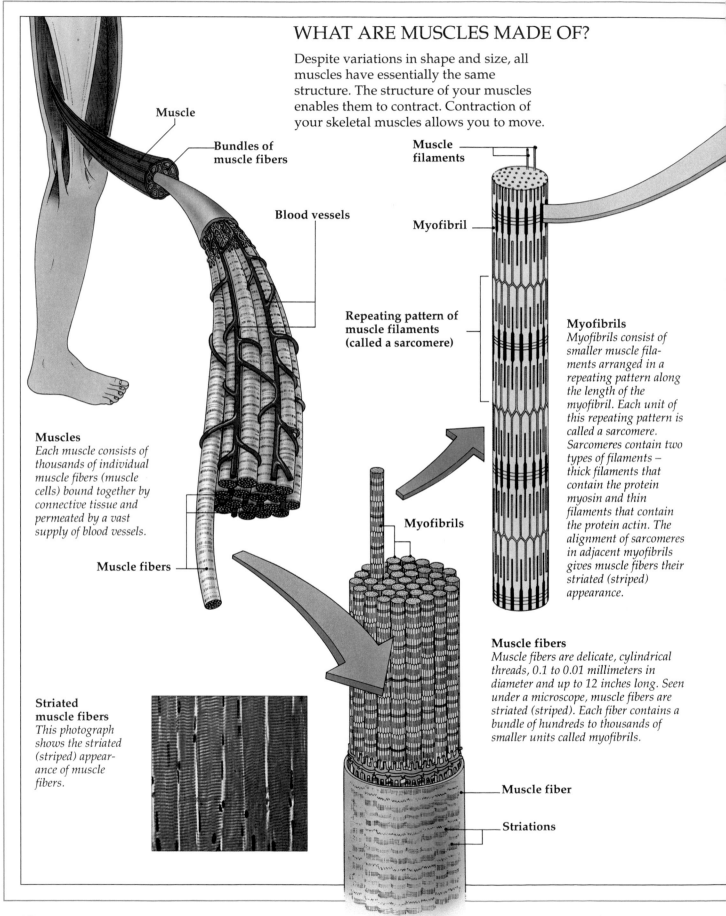

Muscle

Bundles of muscle fibers

Blood vessels

Muscle filaments

Myofibril

Repeating pattern of muscle filaments (called a sarcomere)

Muscles
Each muscle consists of thousands of individual muscle fibers (muscle cells) bound together by connective tissue and permeated by a vast supply of blood vessels.

Muscle fibers

Myofibrils

Myofibrils
Myofibrils consist of smaller muscle filaments arranged in a repeating pattern along the length of the myofibril. Each unit of this repeating pattern is called a sarcomere. Sarcomeres contain two types of filaments – thick filaments that contain the protein myosin and thin filaments that contain the protein actin. The alignment of sarcomeres in adjacent myofibrils gives muscle fibers their striated (striped) appearance.

Muscle fibers
Muscle fibers are delicate, cylindrical threads, 0.1 to 0.01 millimeters in diameter and up to 12 inches long. Seen under a microscope, muscle fibers are striated (striped). Each fiber contains a bundle of hundreds to thousands of smaller units called myofibrils.

Striated muscle fibers
This photograph shows the striated (striped) appearance of muscle fibers.

Muscle fiber

Striations

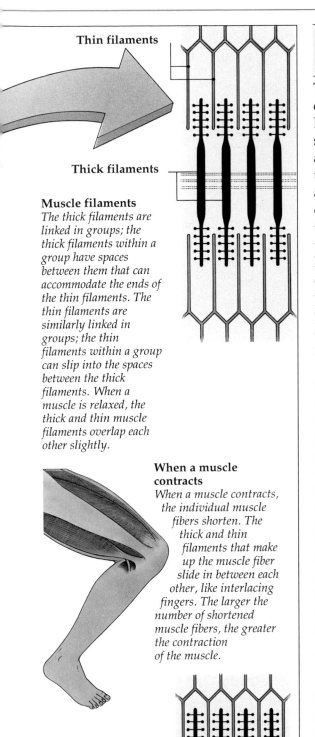

Thin filaments

Thick filaments

Muscle filaments
The thick filaments are linked in groups; the thick filaments within a group have spaces between them that can accommodate the ends of the thin filaments. The thin filaments are similarly linked in groups; the thin filaments within a group can slip into the spaces between the thick filaments. When a muscle is relaxed, the thick and thin muscle filaments overlap each other slightly.

When a muscle contracts
When a muscle contracts, the individual muscle fibers shorten. The thick and thin filaments that make up the muscle fiber slide in between each other, like interlacing fingers. The larger the number of shortened muscle fibers, the greater the contraction of the muscle.

Thick and thin filaments slide in between each other

HOW MUSCLES CAUSE MOVEMENT

There are three types of muscle actions – concentric, eccentric, and isometric. During concentric action, the muscle shortens to produce movement. An example of this is lifting an object from a table. The biceps muscle in your upper arm shortens to perform the movement of lifting. The biceps muscle is also used to lower the object back to the table. In this movement, the biceps muscle is lengthening as it creates force. This is called an eccentric muscle action. When you hold a bag of groceries in your arms, your muscles are producing force without either shortening or lengthening. This is called an isometric muscle action.

Inside your muscle fibers, strands of filaments link together and interact to exert force. In a concentric muscle action (lifting an object), the filaments exert a pull and cause the muscle to shorten. In an eccentric muscle action (lowering an object), the filaments pull against each other in order to resist the lengthening movement. If these filaments were not exerting a pull, you would drop the object. During an isometric muscle action (holding the groceries), the filaments pull and try to shorten but the muscles are fixed in place. The pulling of the filaments against each other provides the necessary tension to hold the bag of groceries.

What stimulates muscle contraction?

Nerve cells (called neurons) in the brain and spinal cord send signals to muscles to cause them to contract. The signals pass down motor neurons (nerve cells that stimulate muscle) that travel from the spinal cord to muscle fibers.

Each motor neuron connects to several muscle fibers. When the signal reaches a muscle fiber, it causes the muscle fiber to shorten. The number of muscle fibers that are shortened determines the force of a movement.

WHAT ARE TENDONS?

Tendons are strong, white cords of fibrous connective tissue that attach skeletal muscles to bones. The slight elasticity of tendons protects muscles and ligaments from excessive strain. The tendon attached to the origin of a muscle (usually the stationary end) is usually fairly short and binds the muscle firmly to the bone. The tendon attached to the insertion end of a muscle (usually the movable end) is often very long. For example, many of the muscles that move your hand and fingers are in the lower part of your arm and are connected to your hand by long tendons that run across the front and back of your wrist.

YOUR JOINTS

Joints are the points at which two or more bones join. The ends of the bones are bound together by fibrous cords called ligaments. Different joints have varying ranges of movement. Freely movable joints are lubricated by the synovial fluid secreted inside the joint and are called synovial joints. The shape of these joints is related to their ranges of movement. Examples of synovial joints are the joints of the shoulders, hips, elbows, and fingers. In slightly movable

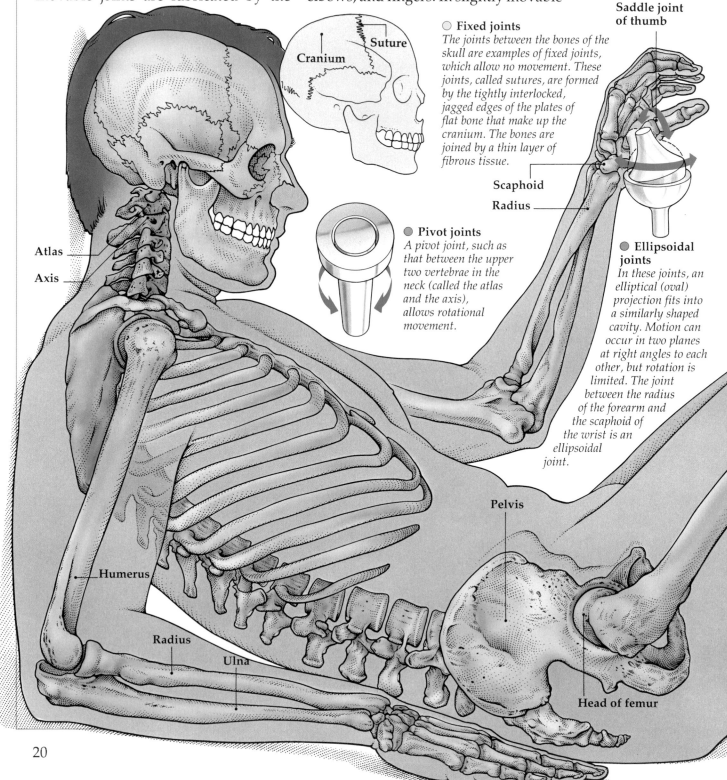

○ **Fixed joints**
The joints between the bones of the skull are examples of fixed joints, which allow no movement. These joints, called sutures, are formed by the tightly interlocked, jagged edges of the plates of flat bone that make up the cranium. The bones are joined by a thin layer of fibrous tissue.

Saddle joint of thumb

Suture

Cranium

Scaphoid

Radius

● **Pivot joints**
A pivot joint, such as that between the upper two vertebrae in the neck (called the atlas and the axis), allows rotational movement.

● **Ellipsoidal joints**
In these joints, an elliptical (oval) projection fits into a similarly shaped cavity. Motion can occur in two planes at right angles to each other, but rotation is limited. The joint between the radius of the forearm and the scaphoid of the wrist is an ellipsoidal joint.

Atlas

Axis

Humerus

Radius

Ulna

Pelvis

Head of femur

joints, fibrous attachments – either ligaments or fibrocartilage (see WHAT IS CARTILAGE? on page 23) – limit the range of movement. Examples of slightly movable joints are those between the vertebrae. Fixed joints, such as the joints between the bones of some parts of the skull, allow no movement. The range of movement of a joint usually relates to the function of the body part that it moves. For example, the relatively free movement of your finger joints allows you to hold a pen and write or to play the piano. The more limited movement of the spinal joints allows you to maintain an upright posture without expending much muscle power.

Saddle joint

The only saddle joint in the body is the joint at the lowest part of the thumb where the thumb is joined to the hand. Each joint surface is convex in one direction and concave in the other; the surfaces are arranged so that they fit together. This kind of joint allows free movement of the thumb except for twisting on its long axis.

Metatarsal-phalangeal joint

Gliding joints

In a gliding joint, the bone surfaces are almost flat. The bones are held together by ligaments so that any rotation of the bones is prevented. Examples of gliding joints are the metatarsal-phalangeal joints between the bones of the foot and the sterno-clavicular joint between the sternum (breastbone) and the clavicles (collarbones).

Hinge joints

In a hinge joint, a curved, convex surface fits into, and rotates within, a curved, concave surface. This kind of joint allows movement in only one plane (forward and backward). The small joints in the fingers and the knee joints are hinge joints. The elbow joint, between the humerus in the upper part of the arm and the radius and ulna in the forearm, is a modified hinge joint. This joint is capable of pivoting as well as hinge movement.

KEY

- Synovial joints
- Slightly movable joints
- ○ Fixed joints

Slightly movable joints

In some slightly movable joints, the bones are secured by short, dense ligaments called interosseous ligaments. One example is the joint between the sides of the tibia and the fibula (the bones of the lower part of the leg). In other slightly movable joints, such as the joints between the vertebrae, the bones are held together by a pad of fibrocartilage.

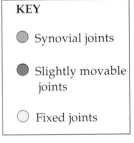

Interosseous ligaments

Fibula

Tibia

Ball-and-socket joints

Examples of ball-and-socket joints are the hip and shoulder joints. At the hip, the almost spherical head of the femur (thighbone) fits into a deep, hemispherical cavity in the pelvis. At the shoulder joint, the rounded head of the humerus (the bone in the upper part of the arm) fits into a cavity in the scapula (shoulder blade). Ball-and-socket joints provide the widest ranges of movement of all joints.

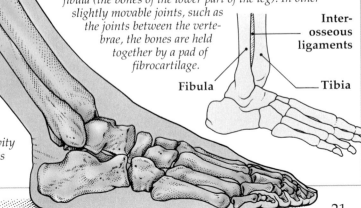

THE STRUCTURE OF A JOINT

Many of the joints in your body are synovial (freely movable) joints. These joints enable you to move your head and limbs and perform a vast range of activities – from running to intricate hand movements. Skeletal muscles attached across the bones that form a joint generate these movements. Despite the different types of synovial joints, all these joints have the same basic structural features, as shown in this illustration of a knee joint. Some features that are specific to the knee joint are also described.

Articular cartilage
The surfaces of bone that form a joint are covered with a firmly bound layer of cartilage called the articular cartilage. This hard-wearing material, when lubricated by synovial fluid, forms a smooth gliding surface. Articular cartilage has the capacity for repair and regeneration in response to normal wear and tear. However, if the articular cartilage becomes worn away or damaged – by disease or injury – exposure of the underlying, sensitive bone causes joint pain and degeneration of the bone surfaces.

Joint capsule and capsular ligaments
Joints are enclosed in tough, fibrous capsules, which help prevent dislocation of the bones. The outer layer of the capsule is formed by fibers made of the protein collagen arranged in parallel bands over the joint; other collagen fibers interlace with these bands. This arrangement of fibers provides strength and flexibility. An inner layer of strong ligaments (called capsular ligaments) reinforces the joint capsule.

CUSHIONS FOR JOINTS

A bursa is a small sac filled with synovial fluid that is found near some joints. It acts like a cushion, helping to prevent wearing of the structures of a joint as the structures slide past each other. A bursa may be located between muscles, between tendons and muscles, between tendons and bone, between bone and the skin, or anywhere else movement is likely to cause wear and tear. There are several bursae located near the patella (kneecap). Bursae are found near other synovial joints such as the shoulder joint and the elbow. Sometimes a bursa becomes inflamed, causing pain and swelling (see BURSITIS on page 100).

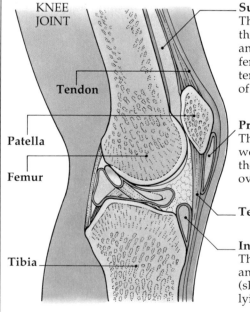

KNEE JOINT

Tendon

Patella

Femur

Tibia

Joint capsule

Synovial fluid
The synovial fluid is a clear, yellowish, sticky liquid similar to the white of an egg; it is 95 percent water. This fluid is a highly efficient lubricant and, in combination with the smooth articular cartilage, allows a joint to move with even less friction than that of ice sliding on ice.

Suprapatellar bursa
This is the largest bursa in the body. It prevents wear and tear between the femur (thighbone) and the tendon attached to the top of the patella (kneecap).

Prepatellar bursa
This bursa prevents wear and tear between the kneecap and the overlying skin.

Tendon

Infrapatellar bursa
This bursa prevents wear and tear between the tibia (shinbone) and the overlying tendon.

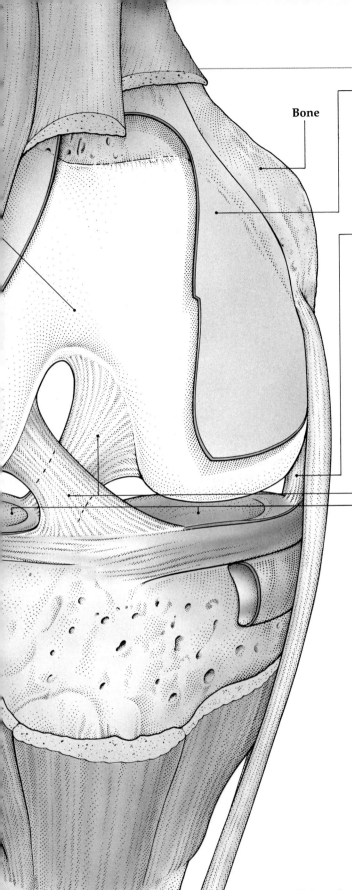

Bone

Synovial membrane
The inner surface of the joint capsule is lined with the synovial membrane. This membrane contains many blood vessels and its active cells constantly secrete a lubricating fluid called synovial fluid. In addition to lining the joint capsule, the synovial membrane encloses and covers all internal ligaments and menisci (pads of cartilage).

Capsular ligament

Internal ligaments
The knee and hip joints have strong ligaments that run from one bone to the other inside the joint.

What are ligaments?
Ligaments are strong, flexible bands of fibrous, connective tissue that attach to bone and usually bind bones together, either tightly or loosely. They are formed from tightly arranged bundles of collagen fibers and have a white appearance. Some ligaments are attached to bone so securely that bone will fracture rather than allow the ligaments to tear off. Most ligaments are relatively nonelastic but some are formed from yellow elastic fibers that stretch to allow slight separation of connected bones. Bones often have special prominences, called processes, to which ligaments are attached.

Menisci (articular discs)
In addition to articular cartilage, the knee and wrist joints also have less firmly attached pads of cartilage called menisci. The edges of these tough fibrocartilage discs are connected to the joint capsule. The menisci act as shock absorbers and as pressure sensors from which information about pressure changes within the joint is sent to the brain.

External ligaments
One or more very strong, fibrous cords run directly from one bone to the other outside the joint capsule. These external ligaments restrict the directions of joint movement. Joints are stabilized by the combined effects of the external and capsular ligaments, the joint capsule, the muscles and muscle tendons that pass across the joint, and the shapes of the joint surfaces.

External ligament

WHAT IS CARTILAGE?
Cartilage is a strong, hard connective tissue that is made up of cells called chondrocytes, which secrete a tough, fibrous, gelatinous substance. There are three types of cartilage in the body. Hyaline cartilage – the most common type – contains fibers of the structural protein called collagen and forms the smooth articular cartilage at the ends of bones inside a joint. Fibrocartilage has a much higher number of collagen fibers and forms the shock-absorbing menisci (pads of cartilage) found in joints such as the knee joint and between the vertebrae. Elastic cartilage contains fibers of the proteins collagen and elastin and provides support in some soft tissues, such as those in the outer ear.

BODY MECHANICS AND MOVEMENT

LEVER SYSTEMS

Most of the bones in your body work as levers operated by muscles. Your joints are the fixed points (fulcrums) around which the levers move. Movement of the forearm bone at the elbow joint illustrates the lever action of most joints.

How a lever works

An example of a lever system is the common seesaw. For a seesaw to work, the weight of one person multiplied by the distance that person sits from the fulcrum should equal the weight of the other person multiplied by the distance that person sits from the fulcrum.

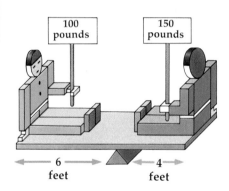

100 pounds   150 pounds

⟵ 6 ⟶   ⟵ 4 ⟶
feet   feet

Your elbow is a lever

In your arm, the elbow joint is the fulcrum. Your biceps muscle, which is attached to the forearm bone about 2 inches from the elbow joint, exerts the pull, or force. Imagine that your arm is bent at a right angle and the distance from the elbow to the palm is 14 inches. To determine how much force your muscle must exert to hold a 1-pound weight, use the formula given above – force multiplied by 2 inches equals 1 pound multiplied by 14 inches. So, to support a 1-pound weight in the hand, the biceps muscle must exert an upward pull, or force, of 7 pounds on the forearm bone.

7-pound force

Biceps

1-pound weight

Fulcrum

Everyday activities, such as walking and lifting, involve elaborate functions of your bones, muscles, and joints. Even the simplest movement requires at least two muscles – one contracts to bend a joint and an opposing one relaxes to allow the movement to occur. Often, for a movement to occur, parts of the body far away from the moving part must be steadied and braced or moved to maintain balance.

WHAT HAPPENS WHEN YOU THROW A BOWLING BALL?

The following description of the body movement that occurs when you throw a bowling ball illustrates how voluntary movements require the coordinated action of many muscles.

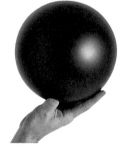

1 As you hold the ball in front of you, the muscles in the front of your forearm contract to maintain your finger grip. The tendency for the weight of the ball to straighten the elbow is counteracted by the muscles that bend your elbow.

2 As you swing your arm backward using the muscles across your shoulder joint, the muscles that bend your elbow relax progressively. Your balance shifts, and the muscles on the front of the spine and in the abdominal wall contract to bend your trunk forward. As your arm and the ball continue to move backward, the muscle tension in your trunk shifts to maintain balance. The muscles on either side of your knees and hips are in balanced tension to stabilize your knees and hip joints.

Trapezius muscle

Latissimus dorsi muscle

External oblique muscle

Greatest gluteal muscle (gluteus maximus)

Peroneal muscle

Anterior tibial muscle

Gastrocnemius muscle

Long extensor muscle of toes

Soleus muscle

3 As you swing your arm forward using your shoulder muscles, your trunk muscles adjust to maintain balance. When you release the ball by relaxing your fore-arm muscles, your trunk muscles readjust to maintain balance.

Deltoid muscle

Triceps muscle of arm

Sartorius muscle

Brachial muscle

Quadriceps muscle

Biceps muscle of arm

Brachioradial muscle

Radial extensor muscle of wrist

Extensor muscles of fingers

Great adductor muscle

Hamstring muscles

Gracilis muscle

Abductor muscle of thumb

Extensor muscle of thumb

How are body movements controlled?

All of your body movements are controlled by the nervous system. The motor cortex (the upper region of your brain) plays a key role in initiating movement. The cerebellum (the small rear part of your brain) is important for the coordination of movement. The cerebellum receives information from the muscles, bones, joints, and tendons as well as from the parts of the brain that are concerned with voluntary movement. This information is analyzed and nerve impulses are sent to your muscles to generate the desired movement.

Many of the musculoskeletal actions necessary for movement are automatic (involuntary) actions. Some movements are skills that have been learned long ago and exercised so often that we are no longer conscious of the various components of each movement.

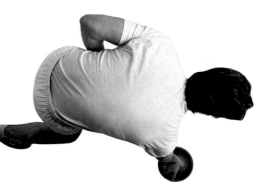

Staying balanced
As the ball is released, the forward force of this movement makes your body pull back with equal force in the opposite direction. Your body needs to be well balanced to provide a stable base.

25

HOW MUSCLES WORK TOGETHER

Muscles are arranged so that the pull of one muscle can be counteracted by the pull of another muscle or a group of muscles. The movement produced by one muscle or group of muscles can be reversed by an opposing muscle or muscle group. When one muscle contracts to bring about movement, its opposing muscle relaxes, resulting in steady, smooth movement. The action of raising and lowering your forearm (see below) illustrates how your muscles work in opposition to each other.

Biceps muscle contracted

Triceps muscle relaxed

1 The biceps muscle contracts to bend the elbow joint to a right angle while the triceps muscle relaxes.

2 When the arm is straightened, the triceps muscle contracts and the biceps muscle relaxes.

Biceps muscle relaxed

Triceps muscle contracted

3 When the arm is completely straight, both muscles are relaxed, although a low level of tension (called muscle tone) is maintained.

Biceps muscle relaxed

Triceps muscle relaxed

WHAT IS MUSCLE TONE?

The natural tension in the fibers of a muscle is called muscle tone. During movement, muscle tone varies constantly. Muscles that are stretched respond by an increase in tension. At rest, all muscles are in a partial state of contraction. This resting muscle tone helps control posture and provide support. Even when you lie down, your muscles don't relax completely. A deeply unconscious person, however, has no muscle tone and his or her muscles are totally relaxed.

Abnormally high muscle tone (or spasticity), which may occur in disorders such as cerebral palsy and multiple sclerosis, causes muscle rigidity and increased resistance to movement. Abnormally low muscle tone (called flaccidity), which may be a feature of disorders such as muscular dystrophy and myasthenia gravis, causes floppiness of the limbs.

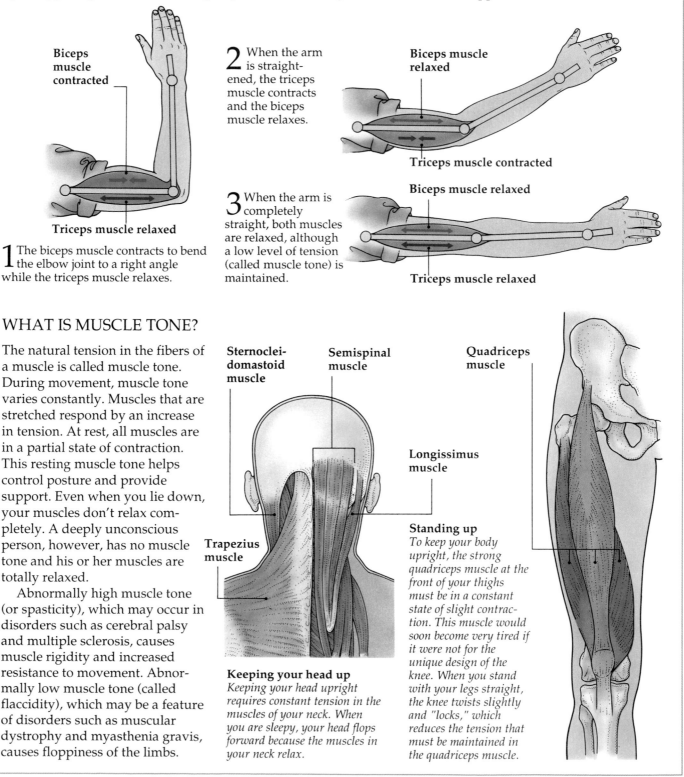

Sternocleidomastoid muscle

Semispinal muscle

Trapezius muscle

Longissimus muscle

Quadriceps muscle

Keeping your head up
Keeping your head upright requires constant tension in the muscles of your neck. When you are sleepy, your head flops forward because the muscles in your neck relax.

Standing up
To keep your body upright, the strong quadriceps muscle at the front of your thighs must be in a constant state of slight contraction. This muscle would soon become very tired if it were not for the unique design of the knee. When you stand with your legs straight, the knee twists slightly and "locks," which reduces the tension that must be maintained in the quadriceps muscle.

THE HUMAN BODY: AN ASTONISHING FEAT OF ENGINEERING

The design of our bodies allows us to perform an amazing range of activities. Animals may be better at certain activities – a cheetah can run at 70 miles per hour, while the top speed for a human is about 25 miles per hour. Yet animals are not as versatile as humans. Our system of bones, muscles, and joints allows us not only to lift heavy weights, run, jump, and perform acrobatics, but also to grasp and manipulate tiny objects with our hands.

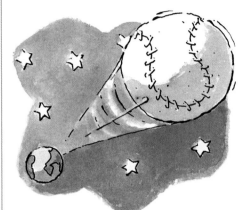

Throwing power
A good pitcher can throw a baseball at 90 miles per hour. The hand, arm, and shoulder all work together. Each component adds to the quickness of motion, so that the ball is released at maximum speed.

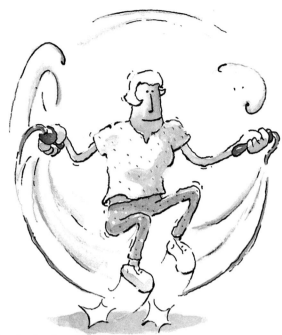

Built-in shock absorbers
Your knee joints and the joints between the vertebrae in your spine have small discs of cartilage that act as shock absorbers.

Strength
Although the entire human skeleton is light, it can support incredible loads. Acrobats who form human pyramids can shoulder total weights of more than 400 pounds. Laboratory tests have shown that healthy leg bones can withstand longitudinal compressive forces of more than 1,000 pounds (½ ton).

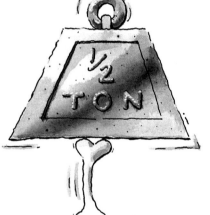

Versatile hands
Humans are the only animals able to touch their thumbs to the tips of every finger on the same hand. This opposing thumb allows a range of grasping abilities that no other animal species has. For example, by wrapping your thumb around your tightly flexed fingers, you are able to grasp small objects strongly. You can also precisely control tiny objects using your thumb and forefinger – for example, you can thread a needle.

Flexibility
The joints of our limbs and trunk allow us great flexibility. Some people naturally have a wider than usual range of joint movement. With training that begins in childhood and regular practice, flexibility can often be increased. Ballet dancers can do splits, acrobats can perform backward flips, and people highly trained in yoga can wrap their feet behind their necks.

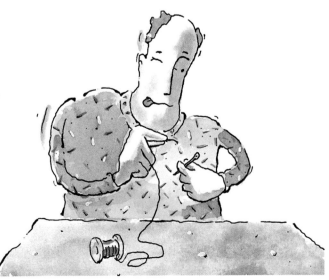

CHAPTER TWO

STAYING IN SHAPE

I F YOU ARE PHYSICALLY active, you are less likely to have minor aches and pains, especially back pain. You have greater flexibility and better posture because of increased muscle tone, and more stable joints as a result of increased muscle strength. Exercising for at least 20 minutes three times a week, on average, can significantly improve your health, physical fitness, and sense of well-being.

While aerobic exercises such as swimming, jogging, and walking mainly improve your cardiovascular fitness (the efficient functioning of your heart and circulatory system), they also have beneficial effects on your muscle strength and tone and on joint flexibility. Stretching and strengthening exercises will help build up the strength and tone of your muscles and will increase your mobility.

A regular exercise program is very important if you are trying to lose weight. The loss of excess body fat that results from exercising regularly – as well as sticking to a well-balanced, low-calorie diet – is beneficial to your bones, muscles, and joints because it reduces the load on the weight-bearing joints of your body. People who are significantly overweight are much more likely to have arthritis in their hip and

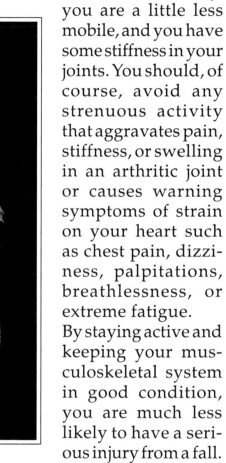

knee joints because of the additional stress and strain that the excess body weight puts on these joints.

Exercising regularly also helps slow down the degeneration in muscles, tendons, ligaments, joints, and bones that occurs naturally as a person ages. It is important to try to remain as active as possible as you get older even though you might find that you become tired more readily, you are a little less mobile, and you have some stiffness in your joints. You should, of course, avoid any strenuous activity that aggravates pain, stiffness, or swelling in an arthritic joint or causes warning symptoms of strain on your heart such as chest pain, dizziness, palpitations, breathlessness, or extreme fatigue.

By staying active and keeping your musculoskeletal system in good condition, you are much less likely to have a serious injury from a fall.

Exercising regularly throughout your life also helps maintain bone mineral density and strength and so reduces your risk of osteoporosis developing. Exercise stimulates the deposition of protein and minerals, creating denser and stronger bones. Bone-strengthening exercise is especially important for women, who become more vulnerable to osteoporosis after the menopause.

THE VALUE OF EXERCISE

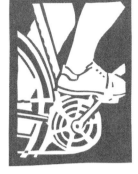

EGULAR PHYSICAL ACTIVITY is an essential part of a healthy life-style. Exercising regularly not only maintains the efficient performance of your heart and lungs, but also keeps your musculoskeletal system – your bones, muscles, and joints – strong, flexible, and more resistant to injury.

When you are physically fit, your body can cope more easily with exertion, both at work and at play. If you exercise regularly, you are less likely to feel uncomfortable or out of breath or to become fatigued after walking up a flight of stairs. Your bones, muscles, and joints are also less vulnerable to injury.

EXERCISE AND STRONG BONES

Regular physical exercise strengthens your bones, making you less vulnerable to a bone fracture and helping protect you against the effects of osteoporosis later in life (see page 36). The mechanical forces on bone that occur during exercise stimulate the growth of bone-forming cells and help these cells work more efficiently. This increases the density of your bones and makes them stronger.

Studies of people who have been inactive for long periods have demonstrated the importance of exercise in building and maintaining healthy, strong bones. The bone density in an arm or leg that has become paralyzed decreases over 2 years by as much as 20 to 40 percent. After this weakening of the bone, the loss of bone tissue tends to level off, with no further significant reduction in density.

Even temporary immobilization such as having your arm in a cast can cause a reduction in bone density. Anyone confined to bed for several months may have a generalized loss of bone tissue; once the person becomes physically active again, the bone tissue slowly returns to its original density and strength.

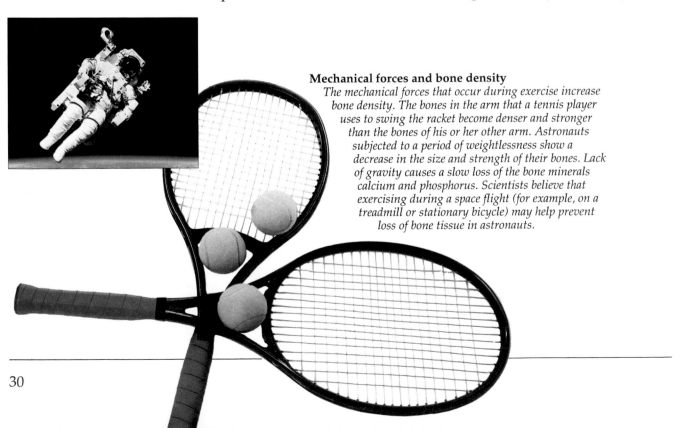

Mechanical forces and bone density
The mechanical forces that occur during exercise increase bone density. The bones in the arm that a tennis player uses to swing the racket become denser and stronger than the bones of his or her other arm. Astronauts subjected to a period of weightlessness show a decrease in the size and strength of their bones. Lack of gravity causes a slow loss of the bone minerals calcium and phosphorus. Scientists believe that exercising during a space flight (for example, on a treadmill or stationary bicycle) may help prevent loss of bone tissue in astronauts.

EXERCISE AND HEALTHY MUSCLES

Regular physical exercise increases the size and strength of individual fibers in your muscles. As a result, your muscles become stronger, contract more efficiently, are less vulnerable to injury, and better protect your joints.

Muscles that are exercised regularly also become more efficient at using oxygen to produce the energy needed for repeated contraction. The following changes occur inside a "trained" muscle:

◆ The number of blood vessels increases, improving the supply of oxygen and nutrients to muscle cells.
◆ A larger amount of glycogen, one of the sources of fuel for muscles, is stored.
◆ There is an increased concentration of myoglobin, a muscle pigment that carries oxygen from the bloodstream.
◆ There is an increase in both the size and the number of mitochondria – the components of muscle cells that use oxygen to produce energy.

EXERCISE AND HEALTHY JOINTS

Loosening-up exercises that move a joint through its full range of motion maintain joint flexibility by gently stretching the lining of the joint capsule and the surrounding soft tissues.

Exercises that stretch the muscles and tendons around a joint improve the mobility of the joint. Muscle-strengthening exercises keep your joints healthy; strong muscles help stabilize joints, making them less vulnerable to injury.

PROTECTING YOUR JOINTS
◆ Warm up with stretching and loosening-up exercises before beginning any strenuous physical activity.
◆ Do not exercise a joint that is painful or inflamed without consulting your doctor.
◆ If a joint feels stiff, don't force its movement without consulting your doctor.

MUSCLE STRENGTH

Doing multiple-repetition exercises using small weights is a safe and effective way to improve the strength and tone of your muscles. It is important to do stretching exercises before and after exercising with weights to prevent your muscles from tightening up too much.

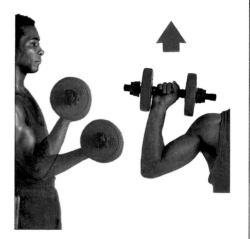

Exercising with weights
Start with weights that are light enough that you are able to do at least eight repetitions. Gradually increase the number of repetitions you do before trying to lift more weight. When you can easily do three sets of 15 repetitions on one muscle group, you can increase the weight.

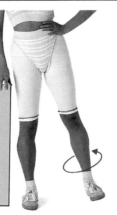

A hip-loosening exercise
Shift all your body weight onto one leg and then circle your free leg from the hip. Start with a very small circle and gradually increase the diameter of the circle as far as you comfortably can. Repeat the exercise, circling in the opposite direction. Then exercise the other leg.

A stretching exercise
While standing, move your right leg back about 2 to 3 feet, keeping your heels on the ground. Then, trying to keep your balance (and without locking your right knee), slowly bend the left knee until you feel the muscles down the back of your right leg stretch. Repeat on the other side. This exercise stretches your calf muscles and the hamstring muscles in the back of your thighs.

AEROBIC EXERCISE

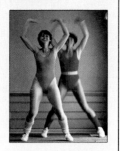

During aerobic exercise, the body meets the muscles' increased demand for oxygen. High-impact aerobics feature running or jumping as part of the exercise routine, while low-impact aerobics involve more upper-body exercises and less jumping. Some fitness experts claim that low-impact aerobics cause fewer injuries. No reliable studies have been done to compare the effects of these types of exercise.

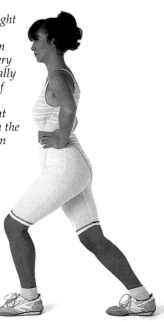

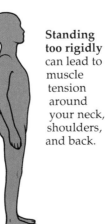

PREVENTING BACK PROBLEMS

MOST PEOPLE have a back problem at some time in their lives. Back problems are usually caused by injury to one of the structures that help support the spine – for example, a ligament sprain. You can help prevent such problems by trying to avoid putting strain on your back and by exercising to strengthen your back and abdominal muscles.

You are more likely to have a back problem if your job involves lifting or carrying heavy loads or if you spend long periods sitting in one position or bending at an awkward angle. The risk of injuring your back is higher if you are overweight, because your spine is supporting a heavier load. In the late months of pregnancy, women often have back pain because the extra weight increases the strain on their spine.

CAN YOUR POSTURE BE IMPROVED?

Good posture consists of efficiently balancing your body weight around your body's center of gravity in the lower part of your spine and pelvis. The correct posture for any activity is that which places the least amount of stress on your back. Exercises that strengthen and tone your back and abdominal muscles can help improve your posture. Back pain is often caused by bad posture, such as slouching or curving the lower part of your back, which places excessive strain on your spine. Any of the habits shown below can lead to back problems.

Standing correctly
When standing correctly, your spine maintains its natural S-shaped curve and the muscles of your back and abdomen are relaxed without being slack. A healthy standing posture is most easily achieved by standing tall with your head erect and your shoulders back. Your weight should be distributed evenly onto both feet. Do not stand with your legs crossed or arch your back into a position that feels uncomfortable.

Standing too rigidly can lead to muscle tension around your neck, shoulders, and back.

Slouching encourages excessive curving of the lower part of your back and a forward-tilted pelvis, increasing the strain on your spine.

Shifting your weight onto one leg habitually may strain the ligaments of that leg.

REDUCING BACK STRAIN

Your spine is subjected to and can withstand considerable stress and strain. Although it is impossible to protect yourself completely against back problems, you can reduce the strain on your back by following the advice given below:

◆ Maintain correct posture and avoid awkward movements, such as bending over and twisting at the same time.

◆ Don't wear high-heeled shoes; they tend to cause forward tilting of the pelvis. This tilt places strain on the muscles and ligaments that are attached to the spine and the joints of the spine.

◆ If your job involves lifting heavy objects, learn techniques that help you avoid injury. Bend your knees and keep your back straight. Make sure the object is directly in front of you and not too far away. Push up from your knees and keep your back straight as you return to a standing position.

◆ Lose any excess weight through regular exercise and sensible dieting.

◆ Exercise regularly to maintain the strength of your back muscles and abdominal muscles (see page 34).

◆ Take time every day to relax. Tension often leads to bad posture and stress-related habits that cause muscle fatigue.

Adjust your car seat
When you drive, the seat of your car should be positioned so that your knees are higher than your hips and you can reach the pedals without stretching your legs. The back of the seat should provide firm support for the lower part of your back.

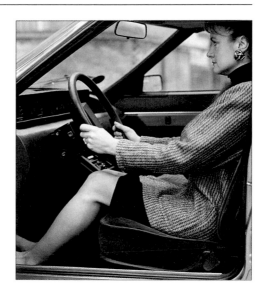

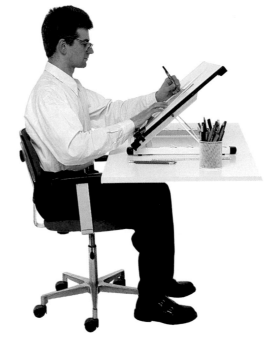

Do you need to alter your work station?
Make sure that your chair has a firm back that supports the lower part of your back. The size and height of the seat should allow you to put your feet flat on the floor and bend your knees comfortably at a right angle so that the seat supports most of your thighs. If you work at a keyboard, the height of your work surface should allow you to sit with your elbows bent at a 70- to 90-degree angle. If you do work such as drawing or proofreading, try a sloped work surface.

Check your mattress
We spend nearly one third of our lives in bed, so it is not surprising that back problems are often caused by a mattress that provides insufficient support. A good mattress is firm, but it need not be hard. If you have been sleeping on a sagging mattress, you should replace it with a firmer one or you can put a board between the mattress and springs.

How many pillows do you use?
It is best to sleep with one flat pillow to support your head. If you want to elevate your legs to help relieve a backache, put a spare pillow under your heels and calves.

EXERCISES TO PROTECT YOUR BACK

If performed on a regular basis, exercises that stretch and strengthen the muscles of your spine can help prevent back problems. If your back and abdominal muscles are strong and toned, it is easier to maintain good posture and keep your spine in its correct position when you are lifting or carrying.

These exercises should be done on a firm surface. Repeat each exercise up to 12 times before you go to the next one, but rest if you feel tired. If any movement causes pain in your back, or down one of your legs, stop doing that exercise immediately.

The exercises shown here are intended only as suggestions. Ask your doctor to help you develop a comprehensive exercise program. If you have a history of back problems, talk to your doctor before performing any of these exercises.

BACK EXERCISES

To stretch your back muscles

Get down on your hands and knees and arch your back upward while bending your head down. Lift the knee of one leg up toward your forehead, then extend that leg straight out behind you and look up at the same time. Repeat this exercise with each leg.

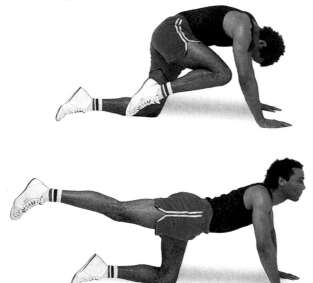

To improve back mobility

The pelvic tilt is the only exercise recommended for people with back problems. Lie on your back with your knees bent and held together and your feet flat on the floor. Push the lower part of your back flat against the floor by tilting your pelvis forward; then arch your back away from the floor. Keep your hips and buttocks on the floor. Finally, raise both your back and your buttocks off the floor and hold this position for a few seconds.

To strengthen your back muscles

1 Lie flat on your stomach with your arms at your sides. Raise your head and shoulders off the floor. Hold this position for a few seconds and then relax.

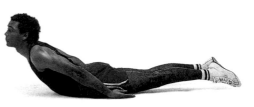

2 Do exercise 1 with your hands behind your head, then with your arms extended in front of you. Do not try to raise your head and shoulders higher than is comfortable.

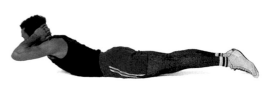

3 Lie on your stomach with your arms in front of you and elbows flexed. Raise each leg in turn, keeping your knee straight. Repeat the exercise, raising both legs together.

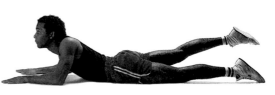

4 Lie flat on your stomach, with your arms extended in front of you. Raise your head and shoulders and, at the same time, raise both legs.

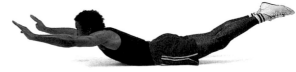

ABDOMINAL EXERCISES

To stretch your abdominal muscles

Lie flat on your stomach, with your hands under your shoulders, palms on the floor, and elbows bent. Push your shoulders and chest up off the floor until you feel a pull across your abdomen. Hold the position for a few seconds and then lower yourself to the floor.

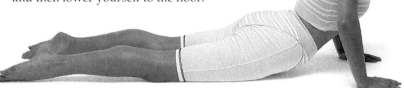

To strengthen your abdominal muscles

1 Lie on your back with your knees bent, clasping your hands behind your head. Pull your shoulders 4 to 6 inches off the floor by raising your head first and then raising your shoulders. Keep your knees bent.

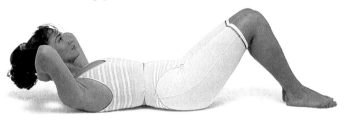

2 Lie on your back with your knees bent, clasping your right hand behind your head and stretching your left arm alongside you on the floor. Without letting your left arm and shoulder leave the ground, move your right elbow toward your left knee as far as you can and then return it to the floor. Then try this exercise with your right arm outstretched on the floor and your left elbow bent.

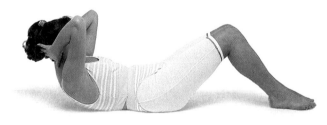

ASK YOUR DOCTOR
BACK PROBLEMS

Q **I frequently have pain in the upper part of my back. Could this pain be caused by the many hours I spend bent over my desk?**

A Yes. It is very common for people who sit in one position for long periods to have pain in the upper part of their back. Try to change your sitting position as much as possible and take regular breaks. If you find that you lean over your desk to work, you may want to try using a sloped work surface. Regular loosening-up exercises to stretch the muscles across your chest may also help prevent your back pain.

Q **Since I broke my left thigh-bone last year, my left leg seems to be shorter than my right leg. Could this be causing pain in the lower part of my back?**

A Yes. If one of your legs is shorter than the other, your pelvis and the lower part of your spine will tilt sideways when you stand up straight. This tilt increases the strain on the lower part of your spine. Talk to your doctor about putting a heel lift, a support, or a brace into your left shoe to balance the difference in the lengths of your legs.

Q **I'm tall and thin, and very active. Even though I don't have any health problems and I'm physically fit, I get backaches. Why?**

A Tall, thin people are more prone to back problems because they have less compact muscles and a longer, less stable spine. You can help prevent backaches by trying to avoid lifting heavy objects and by choosing activities that don't require a lot of twisting and bending.

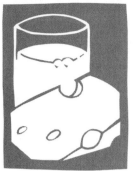

PREVENTING OSTEOPOROSIS

WITH OSTEOPOROSIS, bones become less dense, causing them to become weak and brittle. This loss of density makes bones fracture more easily. During childhood and early adult life, bone density increases steadily, peaking at about age 35. From middle age onward, we all experience some loss of bone density and strength. In women, the rate of bone loss increases substantially for about 10 years after the menopause.

WHO IS AT RISK?

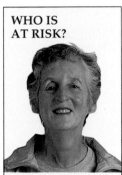

Anyone can be affected by osteoporosis. You are at higher risk of osteoporosis if you:

◆ Are a woman
◆ Are of European or Asian descent
◆ Are underweight or slightly built or have had anorexia nervosa (an eating disorder)
◆ Smoke
◆ Drink alcohol regularly
◆ Have a low calcium intake
◆ Have not given birth to a child
◆ Had an early menopause
◆ Get very little exercise

If you feel you are at high risk of osteoporosis, or if osteoporosis runs in your family, talk to your doctor.

Although osteoporosis is a natural part of aging (see page 58), you can reduce the severity of the condition by exercising regularly and eating a healthy diet that contains enough calcium. Teenage girls and women in their early 20s should consult their doctors about the need for calcium supplements. Hormone replacement therapy can help reduce bone loss after the menopause.

TOUGHENING YOUR BONES

Regular, weight-bearing exercise – in which the bones work against muscles or a force such as gravity – stimulates growth of bone tissue, builds up bone density, and helps delay the onset of osteoporosis or reduce its severity.

EXERCISING REGULARLY

Regular exercise is important at any age. While your bones are growing and maturing (up to ages 25 to 40), regular exercise helps increase your bone density, which offsets the effects of bone loss that occur as you get older. Later in life, exercise helps slow the rate of bone loss.

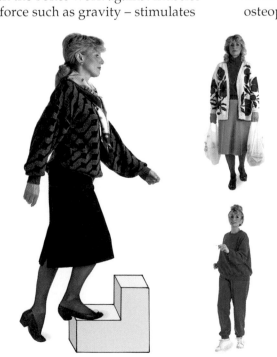

Weight-bearing exercises
The amount of exercise needed to help build your bones does not have to be excessive. Walk to your local store rather than drive; carrying your groceries home from the store is also good exercise. Walk to work if it is close by; make a point of taking a walk at lunchtime. Climb several flights of stairs rather than take the elevator. Several other weight-bearing exercises are listed below:

◆ *Walk or jog 1 to 2 miles, two or three times a week.*
◆ *Dance or exercise to music for 10 minutes each day or for 30 minutes or more once or twice a week.*
◆ *Run in place for 5 to 15 minutes, four to five times a week.*
◆ *Jump rope for 6 to 15 minutes, four to five times a week.*

GETTING ENOUGH CALCIUM

It is important that your diet contain an adequate amount of calcium. This is especially important during childhood and early adult life when bones are still maturing and after the menopause for women. Bones contain 99 percent of your body's calcium. If your intake of calcium is low, calcium is withdrawn from your bones to compensate for the inadequate intake, leading to loss of bone density.

The recommended dietary allowance of calcium for adults 25 years or older is 800 milligrams per day. For adults 18 to 24 years old, the allowance is 1,200 milligrams per day. Pregnant women and women who are breast-feeding need 1,200 milligrams per day.

HORMONE REPLACEMENT THERAPY

Hormone replacement therapy can help minimize osteoporosis in postmenopausal women (see right). It needs to be started very soon after the menopause and continued for at least 5 years. If estrogen alone is taken, it increases the risk of cancer of the uterus, so women who have not had their uterus removed are usually also prescribed a progesterone drug, which eliminates this risk. Women who are taking only estrogen replacement therapy require periodic biopsies of the endometrium (the lining of the uterus). This procedure can be performed in a doctor's office.

Hormone replacement therapy is not usually recommended for women who have had cancer of the breast or uterus or who have a family history of breast cancer. It is also not usually recommended for women who have had pulmonary embolism (obstruction of a blood vessel in the lung), deep-vein thrombosis (a blood clot in the veins located deep in the leg muscles), stroke, hypertension (high blood pressure), or liver disease.

GOOD SOURCES OF CALCIUM

The richest dietary sources of calcium are milk and milk products; dark green, leafy vegetables; citrus fruits; and dried peas and beans. To reduce the amount of saturated fat in your diet, choose skimmed or low-fat milk and milk products. Some examples of foods high in calcium are given below, along with the amount of calcium (in milligrams).

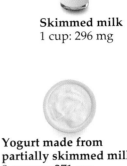

Skimmed milk
1 cup: 296 mg

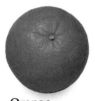

Yogurt made from partially skimmed milk
8 ounces: 271 mg

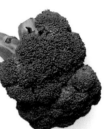

Cottage cheese
4 ounces: 104 mg

Broccoli, cooked
3 medium stalks:
474 mg

Dried beans
8 ounces (cooked):
95 mg

Orange
medium: 54 mg

WHY IS ESTROGEN IMPORTANT?

Before the menopause
Bone tissue is constantly being broken down and re-formed. Estrogen normally limits the rate at which bones are broken down.

Menopause
At the menopause, the ovaries stop producing estrogen. The rate of bone loss increases as the level of estrogen decreases.

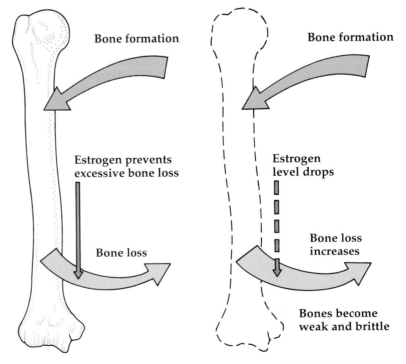

Bone formation

Estrogen prevents
excessive bone loss

Bone loss

Bone formation

Estrogen
level drops

Bone loss
increases

Bones become
weak and brittle

CHAPTER THREE

INVESTIGATING YOUR ACHES AND PAINS

INTRODUCTION

GOING TO
THE DOCTOR

IMAGING BONES,
MUSCLES, AND JOINTS

TESTS FOR
MUSCULOSKELETAL
DISEASE

ABOUT ONE out of every 10 people who go to the doctor has a musculoskeletal problem. For most people, the problem does not require extensive examination or testing. The symptoms usually clear up a few days after resting the affected part of the body and, if needed, taking an analgesic (painkilling) drug. Most of us have had muscle pain after even such simple activities as digging in the garden. In fact, pain is the most common symptom experienced in the bones, muscles, and joints. It is frequently caused by injury or inflammation. Tissue damage triggers the release of various substances in the body that stimulate nerve endings in the affected area. These nerve endings initiate signals that are sent to the spinal cord and then to the brain, where they are interpreted as the sensation we recognize as pain.

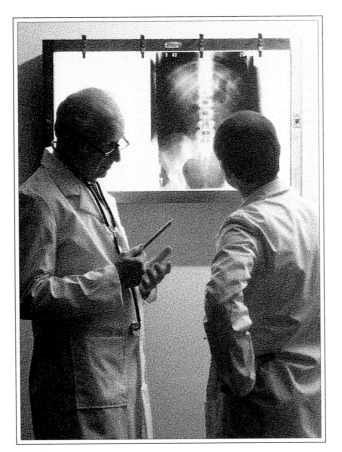

Musculoskeletal pain does not necessarily indicate that you have a disorder of the bones, muscles, or joints. For example, strenuous exercise may cause pain in your muscles and joints. Also, aches and pains in muscles and joints often accompany viral infections, such as influenza, and may occur before other symptoms develop. If you have a bone, muscle, or joint disorder, you may have symptoms other than pain, such as stiffness, tenderness, weakness, and swelling or deformity of affected parts. Musculoskeletal disorders may also be accompanied by general symptoms such as fever, rash, weight loss, excessive tiredness, or a general feeling of being sick.

When you go to see your doctor about a musculoskeletal problem, he or she will decide whether tests are needed to evaluate your condition and whether you need treatment. To make this determination, your doctor needs to know your symptoms, which parts of your body are affected, and the likely cause of your problem. Your doctor will review your medical history and perform a physical examination. In many cases, this will provide sufficient information to make a diagnosis. If necessary, your doctor will arrange for you to have tests to confirm the diagnosis. Some musculoskeletal disorders develop very gradually, so your doctor may need to monitor your condition over a period of time before he or she can make an accurate diagnosis. This chapter tells you about the possible significance of your symptoms, indicates how your doctor will review your medical history and examine your musculoskeletal system, and describes the principal imaging studies and various other tests that may be necessary to confirm a diagnosis.

GOING TO THE DOCTOR

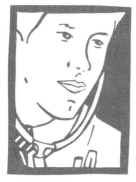

WE ALL SUFFER from occasional aches or pains in some part of our bodies. Most types of musculoskeletal pain are not caused by a serious problem. You often know the most likely cause of your pain and you can treat it yourself with an analgesic such as aspirin. However, there are some situations when it is advisable or essential that you consult your doctor.

Call your doctor immediately if you are in severe pain, if you suspect you may have a broken bone, or if you have symptoms that suggest damage to nerves or blood vessels (such as numbness, tingling, or muscle weakness). If you have swelling, redness, and tenderness that have persisted for more than a few hours and are not starting to get better, you should call your doctor.

YOUR SYMPTOMS AND MEDICAL HISTORY

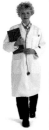

When you go to see your doctor about a persistent or recurrent pain in one of your bones, muscles, or joints, he or she will ask you to describe the aches and pains. Be sure to tell your doctor whether the pain started after an injury and whether you have any other symptoms. Your doctor will also take a detailed medical history, asking you questions about other illnesses and medical conditions.

This information often helps your doctor make a diagnosis, determine which parts of your body need a thorough examination, and decide what tests may be required to confirm a diagnosis. Your doctor may ask you the following questions:

IF YOU HAVE JOINT PAIN, SWELLING, AND STIFFNESS

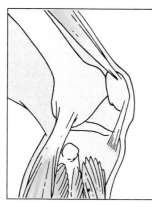

1. How many joints are affected by pain, swelling, and stiffness?

If only one of your joints is affected, you have monarthritis (gout is a type of monarthritis).

If more than one joint is affected, you have polyarthritis. Types of polyarthritis include rheumatoid arthritis (which mainly affects small joints of your hands or feet) and osteoarthritis (which affects a few large joints at random).

2. How long does the joint stiffness remain after you get out of bed in the morning?

If your joints feel stiff in the early morning and take a few hours to loosen up, you may have an inflammatory type of joint disease such as rheumatoid arthritis.

If you have only mild stiffness in the early morning, lasting from 5 to 30 minutes, that is relieved by taking a warm shower, you may have osteoarthritis.

3. Is pain in your joints your most prominent symptom and does the pain seem to worsen toward the end of the day?

If so, you may have a degenerative joint disorder such as osteoarthritis or traumatic arthritis (a form of arthritis that develops in a joint that has been injured).

4. If a recent injury caused your symptoms, how soon after the injury did the swelling begin to become apparent?

If the swelling did not appear for several hours, you may have minor damage to cartilage or a meniscus (a pad of cartilage found in some joints), structures that have a poor or limited blood supply.

If the swelling developed rapidly (within an hour), you may have more serious damage, such as a torn ligament, cartilage, or muscle. Fluid may be produced by the synovial membrane or blood may be spreading from torn vessels.

IF YOU HAVE BACK PAIN AND/OR STIFFNESS

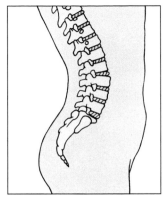

1. Did your back pain begin suddenly or gradually?

If it began suddenly, your pain may be due to a strain on the muscles or ligaments in your back, caused by lifting a heavy object.

If it began gradually, your pain may be due to a problem affecting the mechanics of a joint caused by bad posture or may be due to a disease affecting the joints between the vertebrae in your spine.

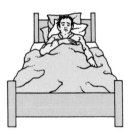

2. Are your symptoms aggravated or relieved by bed rest?

If your back pain and/or stiffness are relieved by bed rest, the symptoms may be caused by a strain on your back.

If you experience a long period of morning stiffness and pain, or your symptoms are aggravated by bed rest, you may have a chronic condition such as ankylosing spondylitis (inflammation of the spine and pelvic joints) or osteoarthritis of the spinal joints.

IF YOU HAVE MUSCLE PAIN AND TENDERNESS

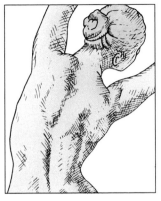

1. Is more than one of your muscles affected?

If you have widespread muscle pain, you may have fibromyalgia (pain in the back and other areas, of unknown cause).

2. Have you injured yourself?

If only one muscle or muscle group is painful or swollen, you may have a muscle strain or tear.

3. In addition to the pain, do you have numbness and tingling?

If so, you may have nerve damage; call your doctor immediately.

IF YOU HAVE MUSCLE WASTING AND WEAKNESS

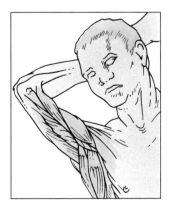

1. Are many of your muscles affected by weakness and wasting (loss of muscle bulk)?

If more than one group of muscles is affected or if you have not had a recent injury, your symptoms may be caused by a disease of the nervous system or of the muscles. There are many such diseases, most of which are rare.

If just one group of muscles is affected, your doctor will ask:

2. Did you injure yourself before these symptoms appeared?

If so, your symptoms may be due to injury to one of your nerves. Recovery will depend on the severity of the injury to the nerve.

IF YOU HAVE BONE PAIN OR TENDERNESS

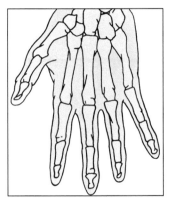

1. Is more than one bone affected by pain and tenderness?

Metabolic or hormonal bone diseases affect many bones.

2. Have you noticed any deformity in addition to pain?

This may indicate a bone disease such as Paget's disease (thickening and deformity of bones) or osteomalacia (softening and bending of the bones).

3. If one bone or area is affected, have you injured that area?

Even if there is no visible deformity, you could have a fracture.

MONITOR YOUR SYMPTOMS
PAINFUL ARM OR LEG

Pain in an arm or leg is a common symptom that is usually caused by an injury. In most cases, arm or leg pain will go away if the limb is rested. However, if the pain persists or recurs, you should call your doctor.

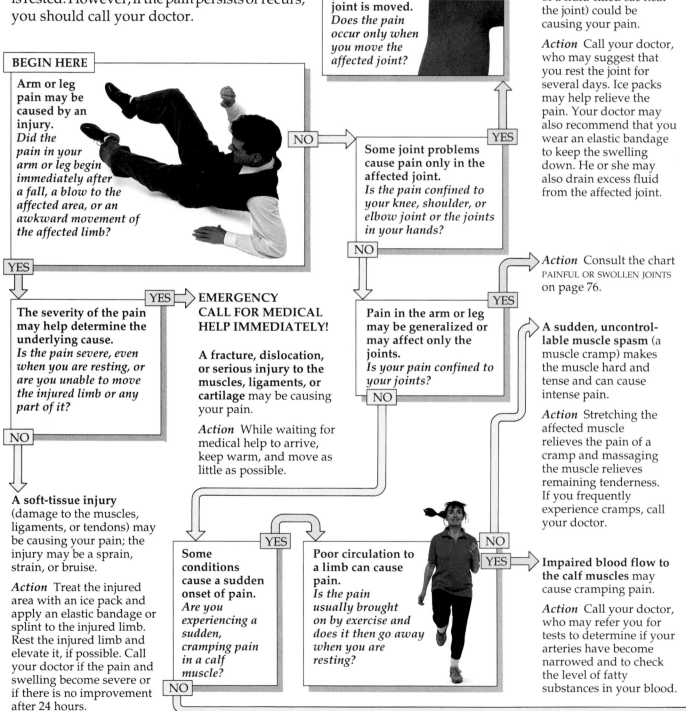

Inflammation inside a joint can produce pain when the joint is moved. *Does the pain occur only when you move the affected joint?*

NO →

YES → **Bursitis** (inflammation of a fluid-filled sac near the joint) could be causing your pain.

Action Call your doctor, who may suggest that you rest the joint for several days. Ice packs may help relieve the pain. Your doctor may also recommend that you wear an elastic bandage to keep the swelling down. He or she may also drain excess fluid from the affected joint.

BEGIN HERE

Arm or leg pain may be caused by an injury. *Did the pain in your arm or leg begin immediately after a fall, a blow to the affected area, or an awkward movement of the affected limb?*

NO →

Some joint problems cause pain only in the affected joint. *Is the pain confined to your knee, shoulder, or elbow joint or the joints in your hands?*

YES →

NO →

YES ↑

YES ↓

The severity of the pain may help determine the underlying cause. *Is the pain severe, even when you are resting, or are you unable to move the injured limb or any part of it?*

YES → **EMERGENCY CALL FOR MEDICAL HELP IMMEDIATELY!**

A fracture, dislocation, or serious injury to the muscles, ligaments, or cartilage may be causing your pain.

Action While waiting for medical help to arrive, keep warm, and move as little as possible.

NO ↓

A soft-tissue injury (damage to the muscles, ligaments, or tendons) may be causing your pain; the injury may be a sprain, strain, or bruise.

Action Treat the injured area with an ice pack and apply an elastic bandage or splint to the injured limb. Rest the injured limb and elevate it, if possible. Call your doctor if the pain and swelling become severe or if there is no improvement after 24 hours.

Action Consult the chart PAINFUL OR SWOLLEN JOINTS on page 76.

Pain in the arm or leg may be generalized or may affect only the joints. *Is your pain confined to your joints?*

YES →

NO ↓

A sudden, uncontrollable muscle spasm (a muscle cramp) makes the muscle hard and tense and can cause intense pain.

Action Stretching the affected muscle relieves the pain of a cramp and massaging the muscle relieves remaining tenderness. If you frequently experience cramps, call your doctor.

YES →

Some conditions cause a sudden onset of pain. *Are you experiencing a sudden, cramping pain in a calf muscle?*

NO →

Poor circulation to a limb can cause pain. *Is the pain usually brought on by exercise and does it then go away when you are resting?*

NO →

YES → **Impaired blood flow to the calf muscles** may cause cramping pain.

Action Call your doctor, who may refer you for tests to determine if your arteries have become narrowed and to check the level of fatty substances in your blood.

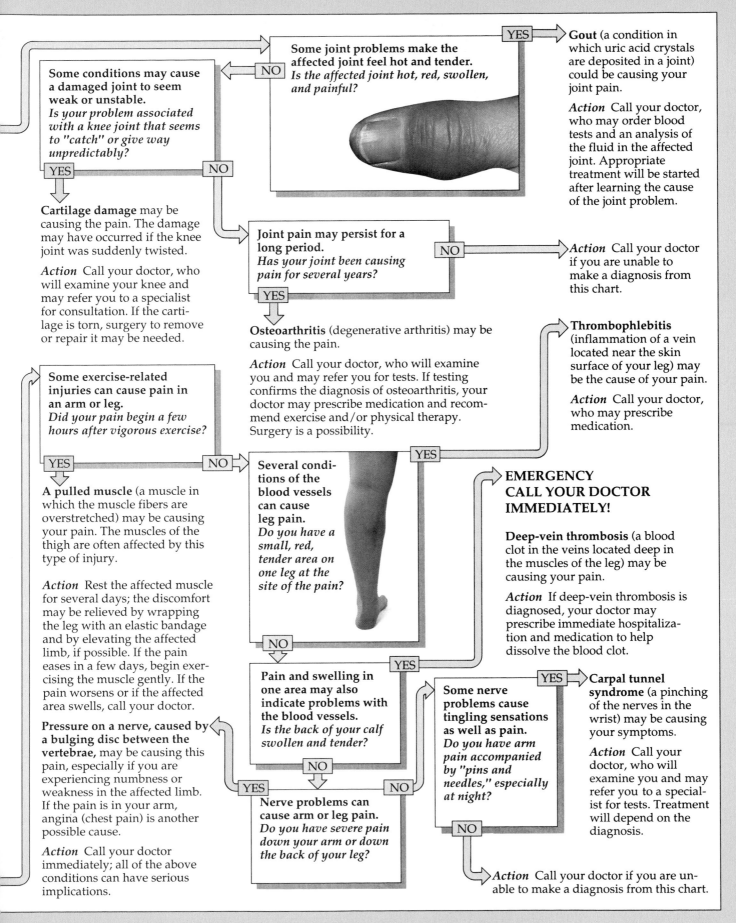

Some conditions may cause a damaged joint to seem weak or unstable.
Is your problem associated with a knee joint that seems to "catch" or give way unpredictably?

YES | NO

Some joint problems make the affected joint feel hot and tender.
Is the affected joint hot, red, swollen, and painful?

NO

YES → **Gout** (a condition in which uric acid crystals are deposited in a joint) could be causing your joint pain.

Action Call your doctor, who may order blood tests and an analysis of the fluid in the affected joint. Appropriate treatment will be started after learning the cause of the joint problem.

Cartilage damage may be causing the pain. The damage may have occurred if the knee joint was suddenly twisted.

Action Call your doctor, who will examine your knee and may refer you to a specialist for consultation. If the cartilage is torn, surgery to remove or repair it may be needed.

Joint pain may persist for a long period.
Has your joint been causing pain for several years?

NO → *Action* Call your doctor if you are unable to make a diagnosis from this chart.

YES

Osteoarthritis (degenerative arthritis) may be causing the pain.

Action Call your doctor, who will examine you and may refer you for tests. If testing confirms the diagnosis of osteoarthritis, your doctor may prescribe medication and recommend exercise and/or physical therapy. Surgery is a possibility.

Some exercise-related injuries can cause pain in an arm or leg.
Did your pain begin a few hours after vigorous exercise?

YES | NO

A pulled muscle (a muscle in which the muscle fibers are overstretched) may be causing your pain. The muscles of the thigh are often affected by this type of injury.

Action Rest the affected muscle for several days; the discomfort may be relieved by wrapping the leg with an elastic bandage and by elevating the affected limb, if possible. If the pain eases in a few days, begin exercising the muscle gently. If the pain worsens or if the affected area swells, call your doctor.

Pressure on a nerve, caused by a bulging disc between the vertebrae, may be causing this pain, especially if you are experiencing numbness or weakness in the affected limb. If the pain is in your arm, angina (chest pain) is another possible cause.

Action Call your doctor immediately; all of the above conditions can have serious implications.

Several conditions of the blood vessels can cause leg pain.
Do you have a small, red, tender area on one leg at the site of the pain?

YES → **Thrombophlebitis** (inflammation of a vein located near the skin surface of your leg) may be the cause of your pain.

Action Call your doctor, who may prescribe medication.

NO

Pain and swelling in one area may also indicate problems with the blood vessels.
Is the back of your calf swollen and tender?

YES → **EMERGENCY CALL YOUR DOCTOR IMMEDIATELY!**

Deep-vein thrombosis (a blood clot in the veins located deep in the muscles of the leg) may be causing your pain.

Action If deep-vein thrombosis is diagnosed, your doctor may prescribe immediate hospitalization and medication to help dissolve the blood clot.

NO

Nerve problems can cause arm or leg pain.
Do you have severe pain down your arm or down the back of your leg?

YES | NO

Some nerve problems cause tingling sensations as well as pain.
Do you have arm pain accompanied by "pins and needles," especially at night?

YES → **Carpal tunnel syndrome** (a pinching of the nerves in the wrist) may be causing your symptoms.

Action Call your doctor, who will examine you and may refer you to a specialist for tests. Treatment will depend on the diagnosis.

NO

Action Call your doctor if you are unable to make a diagnosis from this chart.

PHYSICAL EXAMINATION

Your description of your symptoms and medical history help the doctor determine what parts of your body need to be examined. It also helps him or her make a diagnosis. Your doctor will perform a general physical examination and then carefully examine your entire musculoskeletal system.

EXAMINING YOUR JOINTS

If you have been injured, your doctor will examine the specific joint or joints affected. He or she will also examine other, unaffected joints for comparison with the injured joint. If your doctor suspects that you have a generalized disorder, such as rheumatoid arthritis, he or she will examine all your joints to determine how many are affected and to compare the range of motion between different joints. Your doctor will record the range of motion for all your joints so that any improvement or deterioration in your condition that occurs between this and your next examination can be measured and the success of the treatment you are receiving can be evaluated.

Looking at a joint
Your doctor will look at the overall shape and contour of the joint for any swelling or deformity. He or she also checks the color of the skin. Reddening of the skin, as shown here, is a sign of inflammation.

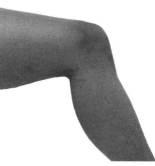

Feeling a joint
Your doctor will feel the skin covering the joint to see if it is warmer than the skin nearby, which is a sign of inflammation. Your doctor will also check for tender areas that could be signs of inflammation or of bone, ligament, or cartilage damage.

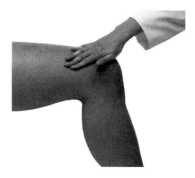

TESTING JOINT MOVEMENT AND STABILITY

Observing your movements
When testing your joints, your doctor asks you to move each joint through its full range of motion, while he or she observes if these movements cause pain and if the movements are restricted.

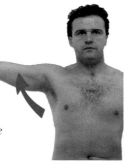

Feeling for "crackling"
While you are moving your joint through its range of motion, your doctor places the palm of his or her hand against the joint to feel for signs of crepitus, a crackling sensation caused by damage to the cartilage surfaces.

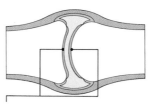

Healthy, smooth cartilage   Worn cartilage

Testing for stiffness
To check for stiffness in a joint, your doctor holds the joint on either side and gently but firmly repeats the series of movements as far as any pain or swelling may allow.

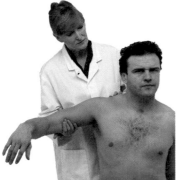

Testing for stability
Your doctor will test the stability of an injured joint by stretching the ligaments in different directions and noting if there is any abnormal looseness.

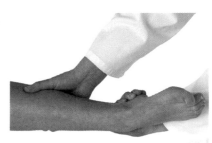

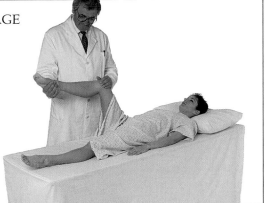

TESTING FOR A TORN KNEE CARTILAGE

With your knee bent at a right angle, your doctor twists the lower part of your leg so that your foot points inward. Then your doctor rotates the lower part of your leg so that your foot points outward; he or she also simultaneously straightens your knee. If this series of movements causes a click that is either heard or felt, it is very likely that the cartilage has been torn.

SIGNS OF INFLAMMATORY JOINT DISEASE

◆ Painful and restricted movement of a joint
◆ Swelling of a joint and surrounding tissues
◆ Reddening and warmth of the skin over a joint
◆ Deformity of a joint

EXAMINING YOUR MUSCLES

If your doctor suspects that you have a generalized muscle disorder, such as muscular dystrophy, he or she will examine all your muscles, checking muscle strength and tone and the strength of your reflexes and looking for a loss of muscle bulk, all of which are signs of muscle wasting.

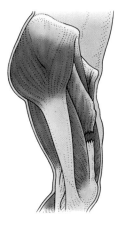

Inspecting shape and contour
Your doctor examines each muscle by looking at its shape and contour. If you have been injured, your doctor checks for deformity that might indicate a tear of the muscle fibers or a hematoma (a blood clot) and feels for the presence of muscle spasms.

Noting skin color
The extent of an injury may in part be reflected by the amount of bruising in the skin over the muscle or farther down the body or limb. This change in skin color represents blood spreading through the adjoining tissues from damaged blood vessels in and around the muscles.

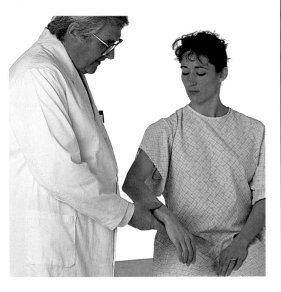

Assessing muscle tone
To evaluate muscle tone, your doctor places his or her hand on the muscle. If the muscle is in spasm, it feels abnormally hard; if there is a loss of tone, the muscle feels flabby.

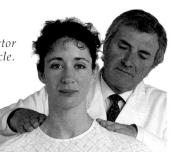

Feeling for tenderness and muscle tears
After an injury, your doctor will press on the muscle to detect tenderness caused by a strain or tear. If the muscle has been torn even slightly, your doctor may be able to feel a gap in the muscle sheath (the fibrous tissue that encloses a muscle).

TESTING MUSCLE STRENGTH

To determine whether a muscle has been weakened by injury (or disease), either to the muscle itself or to one of the nerves that supply impulses to stimulate the muscle, your doctor may ask you to perform strength tests. Your doctor will ask you to move parts of your body on your own as well as against resistance from his or her hand. The strength of your muscles is graded on a scale from 0 to 5 (0 means no contraction of a muscle and 5 means full strength).

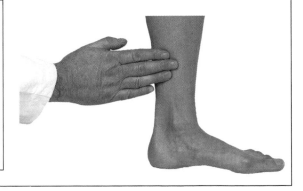

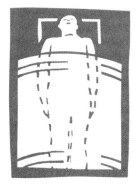

IMAGING BONES, MUSCLES, AND JOINTS

OCTORS RELY on images of the bones, muscles, and joints to help them diagnose and treat a wide range of disorders and injuries. Imaging bones can reveal fractures, osteoporosis, infections, and tumors, which affect the shape and density of bone. Imaging muscles can reveal a tumor or a tear in the muscle fibers. Imaging joints can show damage to cartilage, ligaments, the synovial membrane lining the joint, and the capsule covering the joint.

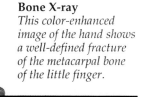

X-ray source

X-raying bones
Having a bone X-ray is a quick and painless procedure. With today's equipment, high-quality X-rays of bone can be produced with only minimal exposure to radiation. However, a lead shield may be used to protect other areas of your body from unnecessary exposure.

Imaging techniques used to look at your bones, muscles, and joints include plain X-ray procedures and those in which a contrast agent (a substance that is opaque to X-rays) is injected into or around a joint or into the spinal canal. In radionuclide scanning, a radioactive substance is injected into the bloodstream and is absorbed into the bones before they are X-rayed. Computed tomography (CT) scanning uses X-rays and a computer to produce cross-sectional images of areas of your body. Other techniques, such as magnetic resonance imaging (MRI) and ultrasound scanning, are being increasingly used.

LOOKING AT BONES

Doctors use imaging techniques to look at a bone for a fracture or to confirm a diagnosis of bone disease.

Bone X-ray

A plain X-ray of bone is the simplest method of obtaining an image of a bone. It is usually the first diagnostic test your doctor uses to establish whether a painful injury is a fracture. You may also have a bone X-ray if your doctor suspects an underlying bone disorder to be the cause of pain, swelling, or deformity. Disorders of bone that an X-ray can detect include osteoporosis (loss of protein and minerals from bone), osteo-

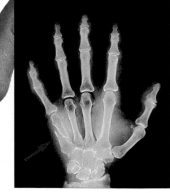

Bone X-ray
This color-enhanced image of the hand shows a well-defined fracture of the metacarpal bone of the little finger.

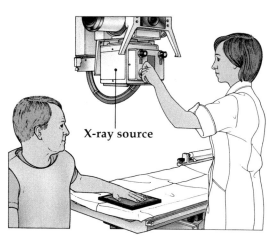

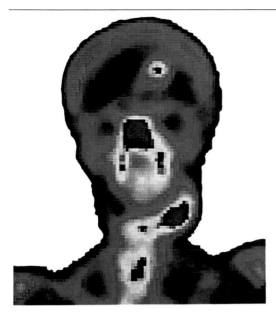

Radionuclide bone scan
This color-enhanced radionuclide scan shows bone cancer (red areas) in the skull and neck. The radioactive substance injected before the scan concentrates more strongly in cancerous bone.

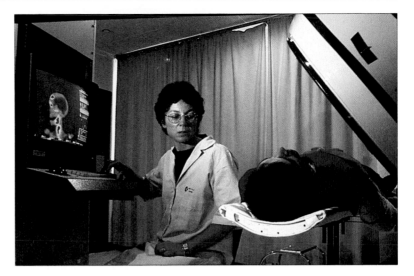

Radionuclide scanning of bone
Technetium, a radioactive substance readily taken up by active bone, is injected into your bloodstream; technetium emits gamma rays that can be detected by a gamma camera. The gamma camera contains sodium iodide crystals. These crystals react to the gamma rays by emitting very small quantities of light. Detectors surrounding the crystals convert the light to electronic signals, which a computer transforms into an image.

malacia (softening and bending of the bones), osteomyelitis (infection of the bones), bone tumors, Paget's disease (thickening and deformity of bones), and bone spurs. X-rays or CT scanning are often used to guide the placement of a needle into a bone to take a biopsy specimen (tissue for laboratory analysis). X-rays are also used to monitor the positioning of a pin to fix a broken bone.

MRI and CT scanning

Magnetic resonance imaging (MRI) is a new technique that can be used to produce a high-quality image of bone without exposing the person to either X-rays or radioactive substances (see page 48 for details of how MRI is done). MRI is used to look at abnormalities of the bone, which include osteomyelitis (see page 65), bone tumors, and aseptic necrosis (areas of bone that have died due to loss of blood supply). MRI is sometimes used in addition to computed tomography (CT) scanning when findings from CT alone are not sufficient, because these two imaging techniques provide slightly different information.

Radionuclide scanning

One of the primary uses of radionuclide scanning is in the early detection of cancer that has spread to bone from other parts of the body. A bone scan may show increased metabolic activity in cancerous bone before an X-ray shows any structural changes. However, false-positive and false-negative results are often produced by radionuclide scanning. Radionuclide scanning is also used to confirm the presence of an infection or fracture in a bone and to reveal a lack of blood flow to an area of bone.

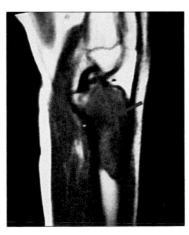

MRI bone scan
An MRI scan can clearly define the size and shape of a bone tumor. The example shown here is a tumor of the tibia, the larger bone in the lower part of the leg (arrow). In cases where a bone tumor is malignant (likely to spread), MRI may enable a surgeon to accurately identify the amount of bone that must be removed.

MRI scan of muscle
The MRI scan below shows healthy muscles of the pelvis and thighs.

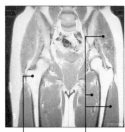

Femur   **Muscles**

LOOKING AT MUSCLES

Imaging techniques are used to investigate a lump in a muscle and to establish whether a muscle has been injured (and, if so, how badly). However, a biopsy of a muscle (see page 54) is the most definitive method for investigating muscle disorders that are not caused by injury.

MRI and ultrasound scanning

MRI of a muscle provides your doctor with information not only about disorders that affect the structure of a muscle (such as tumors or tears) but also about disorders that affect muscle function (such as muscular dystrophy).

Ultrasound scanning can identify whether a swelling is caused by a fluid-filled cyst (such as a Baker's cyst of the knee) or by a solid tumor. Your doctor also uses ultrasound scanning to guide the placement of the needle during a muscle biopsy. Tears of and bleeding into muscles can also be diagnosed.

LOOKING AT JOINTS

Various imaging techniques are used to look for signs of structural damage caused by injury to a joint or to confirm the presence of arthritis.

Joint X-ray

A plain X-ray is usually the first imaging technique that your doctor uses when investigating a joint injury or disorder. It can be used to confirm a diagnosis of arthritis and to help evaluate the severity of the disease in the affected joints. An X-ray can show whether an injury has displaced the ends of a fractured bone. It can also reveal abnormalities caused by arthritis, such as excess fluid, destruction of cartilage, or growth of new bone.

Large electromagnet

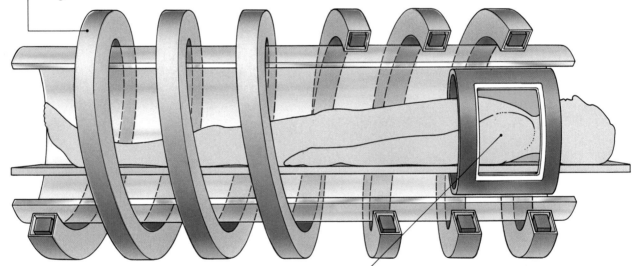

Body area imaged

MRI scan
To have an MRI scan, you lie inside a large, hollow, cylindrical electromagnet. The magnetic field causes the nuclei of some of the hydrogen atoms in your body tissues to line up parallel to each other. An antenna in the magnet aims pulses of radiofrequency energy at the part of your body being examined. This energy moves the nuclei out of alignment. As the nuclei realign, they emit a radio signal, which is picked up by radio receivers inside the scanner. A computer converts the signals into an image ("slice"), based on the strength and location of the signals.

MRI scan of a shoulder joint
The color-enhanced MRI scan at right shows the structures of a healthy shoulder joint. The head of the upper arm bone, which appears greenish yellow, fits into a cavity in the shoulder blade, which appears dark blue.

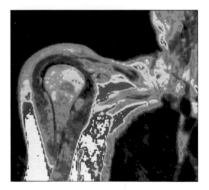

MRI

MRI has become the premier imaging technique for evaluating the tendons and soft tissues of joints. Tears of the meniscus (a disc of cartilage) of the knee or the tendons of the shoulders are shown most accurately using MRI.

Ultrasound scanning

Ultrasound scanning is becoming an increasingly important tool for diagnosing congenital dislocation of the hip in young children. This imaging technique is also useful for detecting an accumulation of fluid inside a joint as the result of an infection or inflammation.

Ultrasound scanning can detect small amounts of fluid and also is used to assist your doctor in accurately guiding a needle into the joint to obtain a sample of the fluid for laboratory analysis.

Arthroscopy

An arthroscope (a thin, rigid telescope) consists of a hollow tube fitted with an eyepiece, lenses, and a light source. The technique of arthroscopy is described further on page 99.

Arthroscopy is most frequently used to examine the inside of the knee joint, but it can also be used to look at other joints such as those in the shoulder, ankle, and jaw. Using the arthroscope, your doctor can examine the surfaces of bone and cartilage inside a joint and make sure that the joint capsule and ligaments are intact. Arthroscopy can pinpoint the extent of an injury and confirm a diagnosis of arthritis. This procedure also has become a widely used method of performing surgery on some joints.

Arthrography

Arthrography is the X-raying of a joint after injection of air and a dye (contrast agent) that is opaque to X-rays. The dye fills the open spaces inside the joint so internal structures can be clearly seen. However, with the introduction of MRI, arthrography is used less often.

Ultrasound examination
An instrument called a transducer is used to pass very high-frequency sound waves into the body. The transducer is held flat against the skin and moved back and forth. A crystal in the transducer converts an electric current into sound waves. The transducer also acts as a receiver, converting the returning echoes into electrical signals. These signals are then fed into an electronic system that transforms them into images that are displayed on a screen.

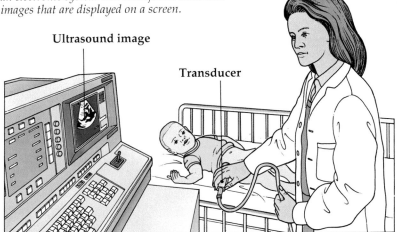

Ultrasound image

Transducer

Ultrasound scan of hip joint
This ultrasound scan shows the hip joint of a child who has a congenital dislocation of the hip – the head of the femur (thighbone) is displaced and lies outside the acetabulum (the pelvic socket).

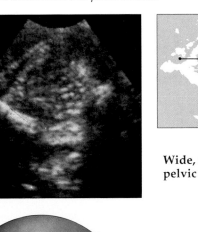

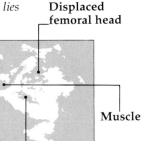

Displaced femoral head

Muscle

Wide, shallow pelvic socket

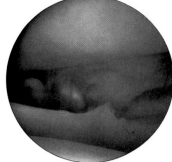

Arthroscopic image
This photograph taken through an arthroscope shows a torn cartilage in the knee joint.

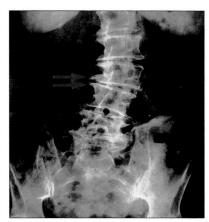

Spinal X-ray
This X-ray shows osteoarthritis affecting the lumbar spine (lower part of the back) of an 80-year-old woman. The joint spaces between the vertebrae have narrowed, the spine has become curved, and the vertebrae have bony outgrowths (called spurs) at their edges (arrows).

LOOKING AT THE SPINE

Imaging techniques are used to look for tumors or signs of structural damage in the spine, to detect evidence of pressure on the spinal cord or spinal nerve roots, and to diagnose or to confirm the presence of other spinal disorders.

Spinal X-ray

A plain X-ray of the spine is usually the first diagnostic test your doctor uses to determine the cause of persistent back pain or sciatica (pain that radiates from the buttocks down the leg). A spinal X-ray can be used to diagnose bone disorders and some joint disorders such as osteoarthritis, ankylosing spondylitis (inflammation of the spine and pelvic joints), a hairline fracture caused by stress on a vertebra, or a bone tumor.

MRI

MRI produces a cross-sectional image of the spine and its supporting structures. This diagnostic technique is especially useful in imaging nonbony structures, such as the spinal cord, discs, nerves, ligaments, and muscles. Using MRI, your doctor obtains detailed images that can reveal damage to the spinal ligaments and muscles. The images also can reveal a disc prolapse (rupture) and can show whether a prolapsed disc is putting undue pressure on the spinal cord or on the spinal nerve roots.

CT scanning

CT scanning is used to diagnose disc prolapse, tumors of the spinal cord, and stenosis (narrowing) of the spinal canal. CT scanning provides a detailed picture of the size and shape of different structures in the spine and the spaces between each of the structures. Abnormalities can be accurately located and the cause of pressure on the spinal cord and nerve roots can be identified. Some surgeons still use myelography (see page 51) with CT before operating on the spine.

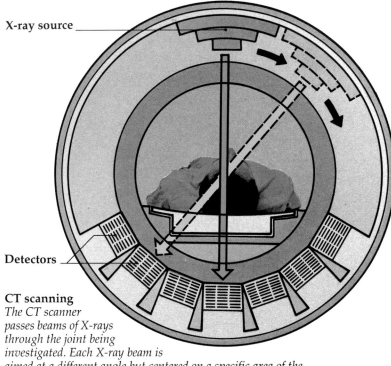

X-ray source

Detectors

CT scanning
The CT scanner passes beams of X-rays through the joint being investigated. Each X-ray beam is aimed at a different angle but centered on a specific area of the joint. X-ray detectors in the scanner record the amount of radiation that is not absorbed by the joint tissues, and a computer interprets the pattern of absorption to produce a detailed picture. The beams create images of "slices" through the joint. A cross-sectional view of each slice is displayed on a screen, and a printout of the picture can be produced for a radiologist's interpretation and report.

Spinal cord   Spinal cord

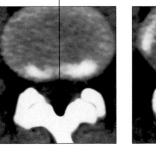
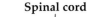
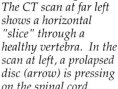

CT scans of spine
The CT scan at far left shows a horizontal "slice" through a healthy vertebra. In the scan at left, a prolapsed disc (arrow) is pressing on the spinal cord.

Healthy vertebra   Prolapsed disc

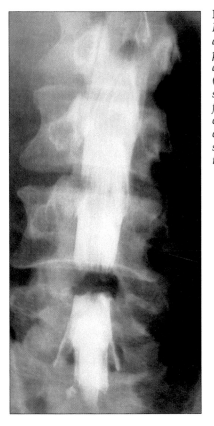

Myelogram
In this myelogram, the dark area shows a prolapsed (ruptured) disc in the lumbar (lower) region of the spine. The cerebrospinal fluid containing a contrast agent does not completely fill part of the spinal canal because of the protruding disc.

Myelography

Myelography is an X-ray technique that uses a contrast agent (a substance that is opaque to X-rays) to produce an image of the spinal cord, the spinal canal down which the spinal cord runs, and the nerve roots that emerge from the spinal cord between each adjacent pair of vertebrae. This technique is used to diagnose a disc prolapse and to demonstrate pressure from a prolapsed disc on surrounding nerve roots. Myelography can also detect tumors of the spinal cord and stenosis (narrowing) of the spinal canal.

Some people have a headache and stiffness in the neck for the first day after myelography. In addition, there is a risk of an allergic reaction to the contrast agent. Now that noninvasive procedures such as MRI and CT scanning are more widely available, doctors use myelography less often for investigating spinal disorders. However, myelography remains a highly accurate, reliable imaging technique and is sometimes used before an operation.

NEW IMAGING TECHNIQUES

The newer imaging techniques provide information about the function of bones and muscles, rather than just structure. These newer techniques produce a pictorial representation of chemical changes in tissues. Until recently, most MRI scanners relied on the detection of hydrogen atoms, which are contained in all body tissues. New MRI techniques based on the detection of phosphorus atoms provide information about the metabolic efficiency of muscle contraction. Other uses for these new techniques are being studied.

ASK YOUR DOCTOR
IMAGING TECHNIQUES

Q I had a radionuclide scan recently. Could the radioactive substance that was injected have any harmful side effects?

A Radionuclide scanning is a safe procedure. It requires only a very low dose of radiation and the substance used quickly loses its radioactivity. However, it is not usually used during pregnancy in order to protect the fetus.

Q I fell and hurt my wrist. My doctor said the X-ray showed no fracture but he put my wrist in a cast. He told me to come back in a week for another X-ray. Is it possible to have a fracture that does not show on an X-ray taken right after an injury?

A Yes. Some fractures, including those of wrist bones such as the scaphoid bone, may become visible on X-rays only after healing has begun.

Q I am 60 years old and have recurrent backaches. My doctor sent me for X-rays. The X-rays showed arthritis, but my doctor says she thinks my pain is due to muscle spasm. Does that sound right?

A If your doctor thinks your symptoms involve muscle rather than bone, she's probably right. Almost everyone over 60 shows evidence of arthritis on an X-ray.

Q My mother's doctor wanted her to have an MRI scan. When he learned that she had a pacemaker he arranged for a CT scan instead. Why?

A Anyone with a pacemaker should not have an MRI scan. The magnetic field of an MRI scanner could make a pacemaker malfunction.

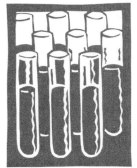

TESTS FOR MUSCULOSKELETAL DISEASE

Y OUR MEDICAL HISTORY, the results of a physical examination, and the findings from imaging studies are the principal sources your doctor uses to diagnose bone, muscle, and joint diseases. In some cases, further testing may play an essential part in establishing a diagnosis. Some tests provide indirect evidence of a suspected disease while others are more specific. The results of a test can also provide information that rules out the possibility of a certain disease.

Samples of blood and urine can be analyzed for levels of various minerals and other substances that have been altered by diseases. Levels of certain proteins in the blood, such as enzymes or antibodies, may also help diagnose a disease. Other tests include a bone or muscle biopsy, analysis of joint fluid, and measurement of muscle or nerve function.

TESTS FOR BONE DISEASE

Analyses of blood and urine samples provide evidence of bone disease. However, in some bone disorders, blood and urine tests are normal. In such cases, a family history and a bone biopsy (see below) can help make a diagnosis.

BONE BIOPSY SAMPLES

A sample of abnormal bone may help make a diagnosis. If a generalized bone disorder is suspected, a sample can be most easily obtained from the pelvic bone. Examination of the tissue under a microscope can confirm characteristic signs of various bone diseases.

Bone biopsy results
This stained sample of bone tissue shows signs of the bone disease osteomalacia. Demineralized areas of bone (stained brown), caused by decreased deposits of calcium, are apparent. Areas of normal bone appear green.

1 The surgical team shaves the skin of the biopsy site over the pelvic bone and cleans the area with antiseptic. A local anesthetic is injected. If another bone is being biopsied, a general anesthetic may be required.

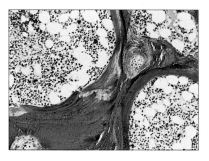

2 The surgeon makes an incision in the skin, inserts the hollow biopsy needle into the bone, and rotates the needle 180 degrees to obtain a sample of bone.

3 Reversing the direction of rotation, the surgeon removes the needle and specimen. The specimen is sent to the laboratory for examination.

4 The surgeon applies a pressure dressing to the biopsy site. He or she then covers the incision with an adhesive dressing.

5 The laboratory technician prepares and stains very small sections of the bone tissue and examines them under a microscope.

Bone-forming minerals

Calcium and phosphorus are important components of bone. In some bone diseases, such as osteomalacia and rickets, calcium levels in the blood and urine are often lower than normal. An increased level of calcium in the blood occurs in hyperparathyroidism (overactivity of the parathyroid glands) and bone cancer. In osteoporosis or Paget's disease, calcium levels in the blood are usually normal.

Levels of phosphorus in the blood are normal in many bone diseases, such as osteoporosis and Paget's disease; however, these levels are low in osteomalacia.

Alkaline phosphatase

Enzymes are proteins that regulate the rates of chemical reactions in your body. Alkaline phosphatase is an enzyme involved in the ongoing process of bone formation. When new bone is being formed, an increased amount of alkaline phosphatase is released into the blood by bone cells. Blood levels of alkaline phosphatase are also normally raised during adolescence and are usually raised in people who have bone diseases such as osteomalacia. The greatest increases in blood levels of alkaline phosphatase are found in people who have Paget's disease (see page 62).

Blood tests
Blood tests are often used to help diagnose bone, muscle, or joint diseases. Levels of sodium, potassium, calcium, and phosphorus may be measured. The levels of enzymes such as alkaline phosphatase and the erythrocyte sedimentation rate (see below) may also be reviewed.

Erythrocyte sedimentation rate
A sample of blood is obtained and placed in a calibrated glass tube. The red blood cells (called erythrocytes) sink to the bottom of the tube, forming a dark red sediment and leaving a clear fluid (called serum) at the top. The rate at which sedimentation of red blood cells occurs – the erythrocyte sedimentation rate – is calculated after 1 hour by measuring the length of the column of serum above the red blood cells. The erythrocyte sedimentation rate is raised in many diseases; therefore, this test is of limited value in identifying a specific disorder.

Calibrated tube

Column of serum

Red blood cells

TESTS FOR MUSCLE DISEASE

A variety of tests for muscle disease help determine whether a disease is due to a disorder of the muscle, of the connections between the nerves and the muscles, or of the nerve supply to the muscle. If the disorder is of the muscle, a biopsy sample of muscle tissue can help your doctor diagnose the disease.

Signs of muscle breakdown

In some muscle disorders in which breakdown of muscle tissue occurs, large quantities of the enzyme creatine kinase are released from the muscles into the blood. In Duchenne type muscular dystrophy (see page 111), the levels of this enzyme may be increased to 300 times the normal value. Less dramatic rises occur in other forms of muscular dystrophy and in some inflammatory diseases such as polymyositis (a chronic disease involving the skeletal muscles).

An oxygen-carrying pigment in muscles – called myoglobin – is sometimes found in the urine when muscle tissue has been severely damaged, which may occur in a crush injury resulting from an automobile accident.

Measuring nerve conduction velocity
Using a stimulating electrode, a small electric shock is applied to a nerve (point A). This causes a nerve signal to travel to the muscle. The occurrence of electrical activity in the muscle (point B) is detected by a recording electrode inserted through the skin into the muscle. The distance between points A and B divided by the time taken for the signal to travel from A to B gives an estimate of the speed of conduction of the signal along the nerve.

Electrical activity of muscles

When a muscle fiber contracts, a brief electrical signal is generated. These signals can be detected by a technique called electromyography (see right). The pattern of these signals changes in various muscle and nerve diseases. Your doctor can distinguish between disorders affecting the muscle fibers, disorders caused by a defect at the junction of the nerve and the muscle, and disorders caused by nerve conduction defects.

Measuring nerve function

By measuring the speed at which nerve impulses travel along a nerve – the nerve conduction velocity (see left) – your doctor determines whether the nerve that transmits impulses to a muscle is func-

Electromyograms of normal and abnormal muscles
The electrical activity produced by a contracting muscle appears as a series of spikes on an electromyogram recording. The upper electromyogram was obtained from a normal, contracting muscle. The lower electromyogram shows evidence of a muscle disease. The spikes are smaller (showing a reduced strength of signals) and show a reduced number of signals.

Normal

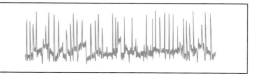

Abnormal

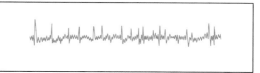

tioning normally. When weakness is the result of a muscle disease, the nerve conduction velocity is normal. In some nerve disorders that cause weakness, the nerve conduction velocity is slowed.

Muscle biopsy samples

A biopsy sample of muscle tissue can be used to detect various abnormalities, such as inflammation and wasting (see below). Abnormalities of the muscle fibers are diagnosed by examining the biopsy tissue under a microscope.

Recording electrode inserted into muscle　**Nerve**　**Stimulating electrode**

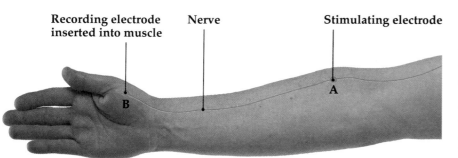

How a muscle biopsy is performed
After administering a local anesthetic, your doctor inserts a biopsy needle into your muscle. The biopsy needle cuts and removes a small sample of muscle tissue. Sometimes a larger sample of tissue is required. In this case, after administration of an anesthetic, your doctor makes a small incision over the muscle with a scalpel, as shown here, and removes a sample of muscle tissue. The biopsy method used depends on the symptoms of your disorder and the suspected diagnosis.

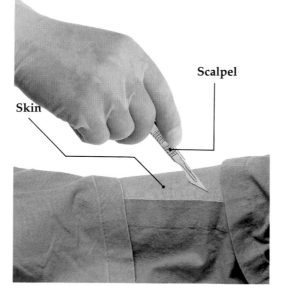

Skin　Scalpel

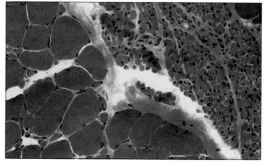

Signs of muscle wasting
This photograph of muscle tissue shows characteristic signs of muscle wasting (degeneration) that has been caused by a loss of nerve stimulation of some of the muscle fibers. The degenerating muscle fibers appear at top right and the healthy muscle fibers are at bottom left.

TESTS FOR JOINT DISEASE

Tests that analyze blood components are used to investigate various kinds of rheumatic disease (pain and stiffness in muscles and joints). For example, the erythrocyte sedimentation rate (see page 53) is done infrequently as a diagnostic test but can be used to provide a general idea of inflammatory activity. Some blood tests that analyze other components of the blood are described below.

Antibody tests

The body's immune system produces antibodies in response to the presence of "foreign" substances. These antibodies circulate in the blood and bind to the foreign substance to destroy it. In some diseases, called autoimmune disorders, the body's immune system produces antibodies against its own tissues. In many cases of rheumatoid arthritis, a group of such antibodies can be detected using the latex fixation test (see right) and other methods.

The antinuclear antibody test is used to screen for systemic lupus erythematosus (a generalized disorder of the body's immune system) and related disorders. A sample of serum – the clear fluid that separates from blood when it clots – is added to tissue such as rat liver, along with a fluorescent substance that attaches to human antibodies. The antinuclear antibody – if present in the serum – binds to nuclei in the rat liver cells and can be identified under a microscope by its pattern of fluorescence.

Uric acid measurement

If your doctor suspects that you have gout (a metabolic disorder that causes attacks of arthritis; see page 90), he or she may measure the levels of uric acid in your blood. Uric acid levels are increased with gout, and detection of uric acid crystals in the fluid from a joint confirms a diagnosis of gout (see top right).

Sampling synovial fluid
Analysis of a sample of synovial fluid may be helpful when examining a joint. A sample of fluid from the joint is drawn out through a needle. If your joint problem is caused by a bacterial infection, the synovial fluid will appear opaque and contain white blood cells. Analyzing synovial fluid for the type of crystals it may contain can distinguish between gout (see page 90) and pseudogout (see page 93). If the fluid contains blood, your joint problem may be caused by injury or hemophilia (inability of the blood to form clots).

KNEE JOINT

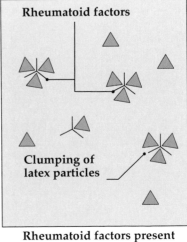

The latex fixation test
This test is often used to detect the presence of certain rheumatoid factors. Rheumatoid factors are antibodies that are produced by the body's immune system against its own tissues. A subgroup of rheumatoid factors can be detected by their ability to cause clumping of tiny, specially treated, latex particles. Clumping of the latex particles occurs in only 80 percent of people with rheumatoid arthritis, so a negative test result for rheumatoid factors does not actually rule out the presence of rheumatoid arthritis.

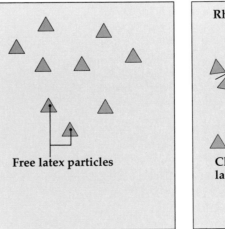

Rheumatoid factors absent

Rheumatoid factors present

CHAPTER FOUR

BONE, MUSCLE, AND JOINT DISORDERS

YOUR BONES, muscles, and joints make up approximately 70 percent of the bulk of your body and provide you with a strong, supportive framework that allows great flexibility and range of movement. Disorders of the bones, muscles, and joints – called musculoskeletal disorders – are responsible for millions of lost working days every year and often also interfere with the normal performance of your activities of daily living. Some musculoskeletal disorders, such as clubfoot, are present at birth. Most, however, develop at a later stage in life. In young adults, injuries are the most common cause of musculoskeletal disorders. Injuries include sprains, strains, and tears of ligaments, tendons, or muscles; cartilage damage; and dislocations and fractures of bones. Other causes of musculoskeletal problems include infection, inflammation of joints, degeneration of bone and joints, tumors, hormonal abnormalities, genetic (inherited) disorders, impairment of blood supply, and attacks by the body's immune system against its own tissues. Your body can recover from many musculoskeletal disorders, such as those caused by minor injuries, in a short period of time; other disorders, such as arthritis, are chronic (long-term) conditions. Severe injury or

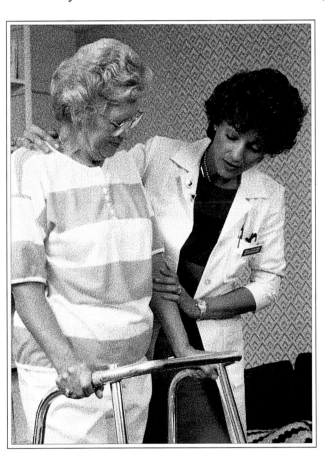

disease can result in permanent deformity. Some musculoskeletal disorders, such as muscle tears, affect only one part of the body; others, such as gout (a metabolic disorder that causes attacks of arthritis in people with high blood levels of uric acid), can affect joints throughout the body. People who have rheumatoid arthritis (an inflammatory joint disease) may develop signs of disease in unrelated parts of the body, such as the eyes, skin, heart, or lungs.

Your sex, age, race, and family medical history may help your doctor diagnose your condition; some musculoskeletal disorders are more common in certain groups of people. Gout occurs much more commonly in men; rheumatoid arthritis is more common in women. Osteoarthritis (a noninflammatory joint disease) and osteoporosis (loss of protein and minerals from bone) are common in people over age 65. Disorders of the bones, muscles, and joints become most apparent in older people. Many, however, do not seek treatment, because symptoms may develop so slowly that the onset of the disorder is hardly noticeable and because they assume their symptoms are a part of aging. Musculoskeletal disorders can often be successfully treated by rest, physical therapy, medication, or surgery.

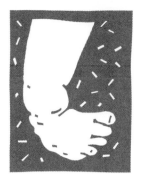

BONE AND SKELETAL DISORDERS

BONE IS A LIVING TISSUE. It is often affected by hormonal, metabolic, and nutritional disorders, such as hyperparathyroidism, Cushing's syndrome, and osteomalacia and rickets. Bone defects, such as clubfoot, are common features of genetic and developmental disorders in children. Some bone disorders, such as osteoporosis, are associated with aging.

In this section, we discuss several bone disorders. For brief discussions of other bone disorders, see the GLOSSARY OF TERMS AND DISORDERS on page 140.

OSTEOPOROSIS

Bones consist of an organic framework on which calcium and other minerals are deposited. In osteoporosis, a reduction in the organic framework causes a reduction in deposited calcium, making bones less dense, weaker, and more prone to fracture than normal bones. Osteoporosis differs from osteomalacia, in which the main problem is reduction in calcium deposition rather than a reduction in the organic framework. The two conditions often occur together, resulting in severe weakness of bone.

Structure of normal bone
Bone consists of an outer layer called the periosteum, a layer of hard, dense bone called cortical bone, and a layer of spongy bone. Adult bone is composed of 65 percent minerals and 35 percent collagen.

Cortical bone — Spongy bone

Periosteum

OSTEON

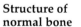

Lamellae — Bone cell

Structure of osteoporotic bone
In osteoporosis, the mineral density of bone is decreased (from 65 percent to between 30 and 35 percent). The layers of bone become thinner and the medullary canal (a hollow canal that runs through the center of bone) enlarges.

Cortical bone — Spongy bone

OSTEON

Gaps
Bone cell
Lamellae

Periosteum

Medullary canal

Structural units of normal bone
Cortical (hard) bone is made of osteons (rod-shaped units), which consist of layers called lamellae. The cells that maintain bone are located between the layers. In normal bone, these layers are packed closely together, as shown above and in the photograph at right.

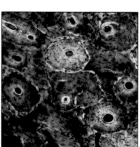

Structural units of osteoporotic bone
In bone affected by osteoporosis, gaps develop between the lamellar layers (above), making the bone weak. The photograph at right shows many gaps (white areas) where bone minerals have been lost.

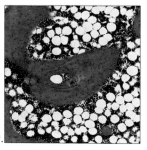

Why does osteoporosis occur?

Throughout life, bone is constantly built up and broken down again. Bone cells called osteoblasts build up bone; bone cells known as osteoclasts break down bone. While bones are growing, the rate of bone formation exceeds the rate of breakdown; by middle age, the rates are about equal. After the age of about 35, bones show a steady loss of bulk and strength, resulting in a slowly progressive process called senile osteoporosis. Because estrogen is important in maintaining bone mass in women (see page 37), the rate of bone loss increases around the time of the menopause.

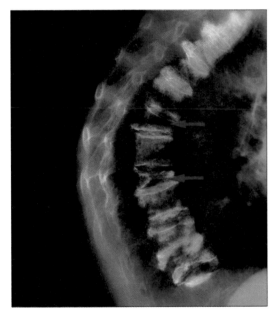

Osteoporotic spine
This color-enhanced X-ray (at left) shows several collapsed vertebrae (arrows) in the spine of a woman with osteoporosis. Outward curvature of the spine has also occurred.

Dual photon densitometry
This is one technique that is used to measure bone mineral density. Dual beams of photons (particles of radiant energy) are directed through the spine (at right). The amount of energy absorbed is related to the amount of bone that the beams pass through. The higher the absorption of energy (darker areas in scan), the higher the density of the bone. The colored bar at the top of the scan indicates bone density.

High density   Low density

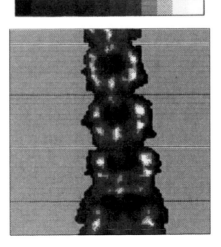

Effects of osteoporosis

The most obvious effect of osteoporosis is an increased tendency for bone to fracture. Fractures usually occur at the wrist, spine, hip, humerus (upper arm bone), and tibia (shinbone). Vertebrae weakened by osteoporosis can fracture and compress, often leading to loss of height and a humplike curvature of the spine. If a vertebra collapses, it can cause sharp, severe back pain, but some people have only a generalized ache. In rare cases, a person may have no pain.

Diagnosis

Severe osteoporosis is often diagnosed only after a fracture has occurred. The diagnosis can be confirmed by bone X-rays. Dual photon densitometry (see illustration at bottom left) can also be used to measure the mineral density of bone. Blood and urine tests and sometimes bone biopsy (see page 52) may be necessary to rule out other bone disorders, such as osteomalacia.

Treatment

Preventive measures can help reduce the severity of osteoporosis (see PREVENTING OSTEOPOROSIS on page 36). Treatment of osteoporosis is difficult, although researchers continue to look for effective methods of preventing further bone loss and building new bone.

Hormone replacement therapy helps reduce bone loss and is effective in preventing osteoporosis if taken just after the menopause. However, hormone replacement therapy cannot replace bone. Sodium fluoride can stimulate the formation of new bone, but bone formed in this way may be weak. Treatment with the thyroid hormone calcitonin has been investigated but this treatment causes unpleasant side effects. Etidronate, one of a group of drugs called diphosphonates, is a drug that has been shown to increase bone density, especially in the spine; however, its role in treating osteoporosis is not yet established.

OSTEOMALACIA

Osteomalacia is a condition affecting adults in which the bones become weakened because of demineralization (loss of calcium and phosphorus). In children, a similar condition is called rickets.

Causes of osteomalacia

The usual cause of osteomalacia is a deficiency of vitamin D. Bone is constantly being broken down and re-formed and needs an abundant supply of calcium and phosphorus. Vitamin D plays an essential role in the absorption of calcium from the intestines and in the reduction of the amount of phosphorus excreted in the urine. Vitamin D deficiency causes blood levels of calcium and phosphorus to become abnormally low, leading to loss of these minerals from bones. Anticonvulsant drugs (used to treat epilepsy) can lead to osteomalacia by interfering with the activity of vitamin D in the body. Osteomalacia may also result from an increased acidity level of the blood and from kidney failure.

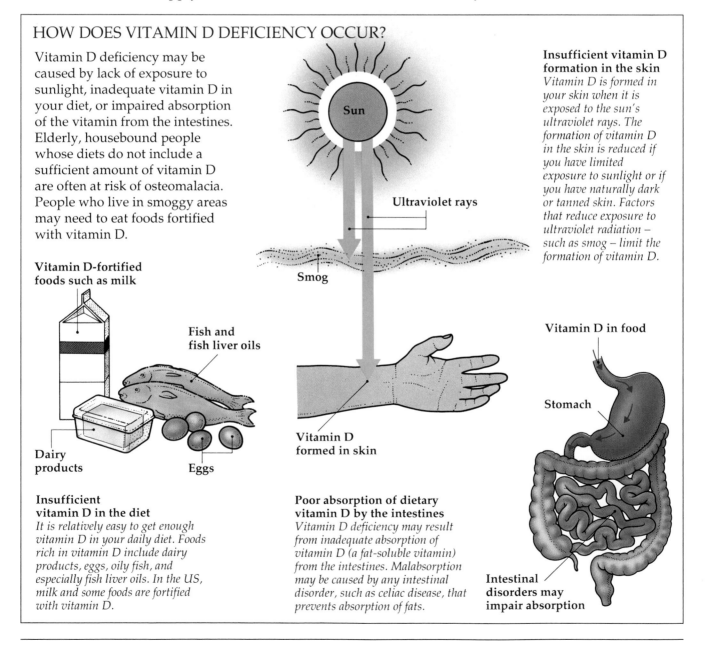

HOW DOES VITAMIN D DEFICIENCY OCCUR?

Vitamin D deficiency may be caused by lack of exposure to sunlight, inadequate vitamin D in your diet, or impaired absorption of the vitamin from the intestines. Elderly, housebound people whose diets do not include a sufficient amount of vitamin D are often at risk of osteomalacia. People who live in smoggy areas may need to eat foods fortified with vitamin D.

Sun

Ultraviolet rays

Smog

Vitamin D-fortified foods such as milk

Fish and fish liver oils

Dairy products

Eggs

Vitamin D formed in skin

Insufficient vitamin D formation in the skin
Vitamin D is formed in your skin when it is exposed to the sun's ultraviolet rays. The formation of vitamin D in the skin is reduced if you have limited exposure to sunlight or if you have naturally dark or tanned skin. Factors that reduce exposure to ultraviolet radiation – such as smog – limit the formation of vitamin D.

Vitamin D in food

Stomach

Intestinal disorders may impair absorption

Insufficient vitamin D in the diet
It is relatively easy to get enough vitamin D in your daily diet. Foods rich in vitamin D include dairy products, eggs, oily fish, and especially fish liver oils. In the US, milk and some foods are fortified with vitamin D.

Poor absorption of dietary vitamin D by the intestines
Vitamin D deficiency may result from inadequate absorption of vitamin D (a fat-soluble vitamin) from the intestines. Malabsorption may be caused by any intestinal disorder, such as celiac disease, that prevents absorption of fats.

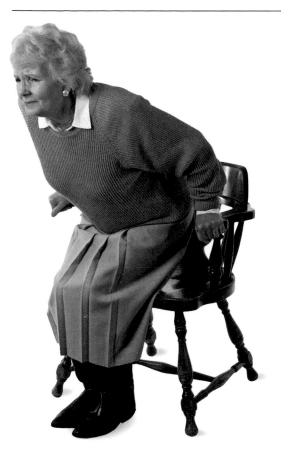

Restricted mobility
People with osteomalacia frequently have a waddling gait because of pain in the hips and weakness of the muscles in the lower part of the legs. They often have difficulty getting up out of low chairs or getting into a car, and may have trouble climbing stairs. Older people with this condition sometimes cannot walk.

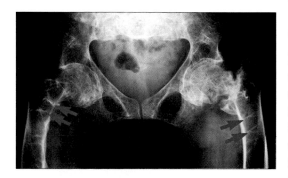

Ribbonlike zones of bone
This X-ray from a person with osteomalacia shows pseudofractures (arrows) – ribbonlike areas of bone that have been weakened by demineralization – in the femurs (upper leg bones). These pseudofractures are a characteristic sign of osteomalacia. The pelvis, the ribs, and the shoulder blades are other bones in which pseudofractures commonly occur.

Symptoms

Osteomalacia causes bone pain and tenderness. The symptoms are often confined to the neck, ribs, hips, and legs. The disease also causes deformity of the skeleton. A person with osteomalacia frequently has difficulty walking and may be awakened from sleep by pain. Mobility may be restricted further by muscle weakness, the cause of which is not known; other characteristics of this condition are described at left. If the level of calcium in the blood is very low, some of the muscles may go into painful spasms, a condition called tetany.

Diagnosis

Osteomalacia can be diagnosed from the symptoms, along with various tests. A blood test can confirm the diagnosis if it shows low levels of calcium, phosphorus, and vitamin D. The blood level of alkaline phosphatase, an enzyme involved in formation and breakdown of bone, is usually increased as bone cells try to compensate and make new bone (see page 53). The level of calcium in the urine is also decreased. Bone X-rays show a decreased bone density and other signs of the disease (see bottom left). The spinal vertebrae may become concave on their upper and lower surfaces. A bone biopsy usually confirms the diagnosis.

Treatment

If osteomalacia has been caused by inadequate intake of vitamin D, limited exposure to sunlight, or both, vitamin D supplements are a common method of treatment. Mobility and muscle strength usually improve quickly. Bone pain may temporarily increase, but the symptoms soon disappear. The person must ensure that his or her diet includes adequate vitamin D. If the condition was caused by a kidney disorder or impaired absorption of vitamin D from the intestines, the underlying disorder must be treated. The person may also receive vitamin D and calcium supplements.

RICKETS IN CHILDREN

Rickets is a form of osteomalacia that occurs in children. Nutritional rickets, rare in developed countries, is caused by insufficient vitamin D in the diet. Rickets may also be caused by inadequate formation of vitamin D in the skin or by metabolic disorders. A child who has rickets may be listless and irritable, is susceptible to fractures, has weak muscles, and has abnormal growth. If the disease is not treated, progressive bone deformities develop. Often the bones in the legs become bowed, in part from the stress of bearing the child's weight. Curvature of the spine may also develop. Nutritional rickets is treated with large, daily doses of vitamin D. This improves muscle strength, helps damaged bones heal, and prevents further progression of the disease. Children with rickets caused by a metabolic disorder receive treatment to control or eliminate the underlying condition; they also require supplements of calcium, phosphorus, and vitamin D. Children who have severe bone deformity may need surgery.

PAGET'S DISEASE

In Paget's disease (also called osteitis deformans), the normal process of bone formation is disturbed. Paget's disease causes increased breakdown of bone and the formation of abnormal bone in its place. The blood supply to affected bone is also substantially increased.

Among bone disorders, Paget's disease is second in frequency to osteoporosis. Paget's disease is uncommon among people under 40 but it affects up to 3 percent of people over 40. Obvious symptoms develop in only about 5 percent of people with this disease.

The cause of Paget's disease is unknown. However, the findings that it occurs more commonly in certain geographic areas and that viruslike particles are found in some bone cells suggest that a viral infection may be involved.

What are the effects?

Paget's disease may initially be confined to a single bone but often spreads to other bones. The bones that are most often affected include the skull, the spine, the pelvis, and the leg bones.

The most common symptoms of Paget's disease are bone pain, deformity (such as bowing of the legs), and fracture. The pain may be in the affected bone or may be caused by complications of the disease, such as a fracture or arthritis in a joint. A tumor develops in 5 percent of people with Paget's disease. The tumor is usually an osteosarcoma (a form of primary bone cancer).

Symptoms and diagnosis

Although bone pain is a common symptom of Paget's disease, early stages of the disease often cause no symptoms. The appearance of people with Paget's disease may gradually, almost imperceptibly, change because of bone enlargement or deformity. A person with Paget's disease whose skull is affected may no-

Bone thickening and enlargement
Paget's disease may cause thickening and enlargement of affected bones. These skull X-rays show a normal skull (top right) and a skull affected by Paget's disease (bottom right). The white, spotty patches in the skull affected by Paget's disease are areas of increased bone density. Enlargement of the skull sometimes causes headache and other problems, such as hearing loss or paralysis of the facial muscles, due to compression of cranial nerves.

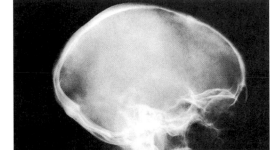

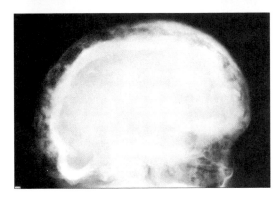

Bowing deformity
Bone affected by Paget's disease has an abnormal, thickened, enlarged structure and becomes weak. This may result in bone deformity, particularly bowing of the affected long bones, as shown here in a person with widespread Paget's disease.

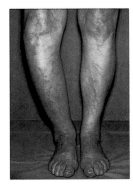

Susceptibility to fracture
Previously undiagnosed Paget's disease is often revealed when a fracture occurs as a result of weakening of the affected bone. Fractures of the tibia and fibula (lower leg bones) shown in the X-ray below have occurred as a result of Paget's disease.

tice that his or her hat size progressively increases. The skin overlying bone affected by Paget's disease may feel warm (caused by the increase in blood supply to affected bone). A diagnosis can usually be confirmed by X-rays, as well as laboratory findings, especially a markedly elevated alkaline phosphatase level in the blood (see page 53).

Treating the disease

Most cases of Paget's disease do not require treatment, although periodic monitoring of the affected bones is recommended. In severe cases, treatment may include painkillers and disodium etidronate or calcitonin, which inhibit the excessive breakdown of bone.

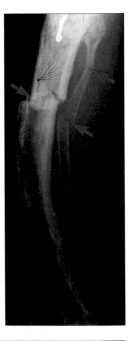

BONE TUMORS

Bone tumors are growths in bone. They may be benign (noncancerous) or malignant (cancerous). When a malignant growth originates in the bone, it is called primary bone cancer. More commonly, a bone tumor is the result of cancer that has spread to bone from another site in the body (called secondary bone cancer). Primary cancers in bone and cartilage represent only 0.5 percent of all types of cancers in the US. However, benign tumors of bone are common.

PRIMARY BONE CANCER

Primary bone cancer is rare. The most common form is osteosarcoma, which affects only one person in a million per year. Osteosarcoma occurs mainly in adolescents and young adults. However, osteosarcoma sometimes occurs in older people as a complication of Paget's disease, when it may develop at more than one site. The tumor spreads rapidly via the bloodstream to other parts of the body, especially the lungs.

Pain in the affected bone and sometimes a visible swelling of the affected arm or leg are usually the only symptoms of osteosarcoma until the cancer has spread. X-rays, bone scans, and a bone biopsy are usually performed to confirm a diagnosis of osteosarcoma.

Chondrosarcoma is another type of primary bone cancer. It originates from cartilage and affects mainly the pelvis, ribs, and breastbone. Ewing's tumor and multiple myeloma are cancers that start in the bone marrow.

Treatment

The treatment of primary bone cancers depends on how far the disease has spread. Many cases of primary bone cancer can be successfully treated by chemotherapy (anticancer drugs) and replacement of the part of the bone that contains

Osteosarcoma
Osteosarcoma usually occurs in a long bone, most often at the lower end of the femur (thighbone) just above the knee. The X-ray at far right shows an osteosarcoma (the hazy white area) surrounding the thighbone, which has become abnormally narrowed. The knee joint is at the bottom of the X-ray.

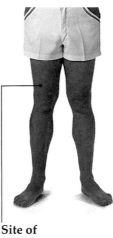
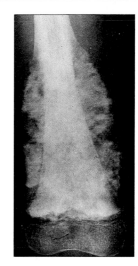

Site of tumor

the cancer with a human bone graft obtained from a bone bank. Amputation is still performed in some cases, followed by a course of chemotherapy. If the cancer has spread to other tissues, radiation therapy is often used.

BENIGN BONE TUMORS

The most common type of benign (noncancerous) bone tumor is an osteochondroma. Other types include osteoma (a rounded swelling that can occur on any bone) and chondroma (a tumor composed of cartilage cells). These tumors are painless and usually require no treatment. If the tumor becomes very large, surgical removal is usually required. Osteoclastomas (giant cell tumors) are another type of benign bone tumor.

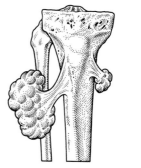

Osteochondroma
The illustration above shows a small and a large osteochondroma. Each tumor consists of a growth of bone and cartilage. The tumor usually begins to develop in childhood.

Giant cell tumor
Unlike other benign bone tumors, a giant cell tumor (right) can be painful. It usually occurs in young adults, often in the arm or leg. The tumor destroys the adjacent bone; at the same time, new bone forms at the site around the tumor. Surgery to remove the tumor is often successful, but the tumor recurs in a small number of cases.

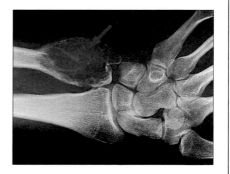

SECONDARY BONE CANCER

Secondary bone cancer, also called metastatic bone cancer, is cancer that has spread to bone from elsewhere in the body. It is much more common than primary bone cancer. Unlike primary bone cancer, secondary bone cancer is more likely to occur later in life.

The most common symptom of secondary bone cancer is pain. Fractures occur and are associated with bone swelling or deformity. Sometimes, cancerous tissue invades the bone marrow. This may prevent the normal formation of platelets and blood cells. Secondary bone cancer may cause an abnormally high level of calcium in the blood, leading to a variety of symptoms such as nausea, depression, weakness, and excessive thirst. A diagnosis of secondary bone cancer is confirmed by X-rays or bone scans (see pages 47 and 48). Secondary bone cancer is sometimes discovered before the site of the primary cancer is identified.

Treatment

Analgesic drugs are usually prescribed for immediate pain relief. Other drugs may be prescribed to reduce the size of the tumor and to treat increased levels of calcium in the blood. Radiation therapy may also provide relief from symptoms.

Specific treatment of secondary bone cancer depends on the nature of the primary cancer. For example, radioactive iodine is administered if the cancer originated in the thyroid gland; therapy with a hormone drug is given if the cancer has spread from the breast or prostate gland. A fracture requires immobilization in a cast and, in many instances, surgery.

The outlook for people with secondary bone cancer depends on the nature of the disease and how far the disease has spread. Some people survive for years after cancer has been diagnosed.

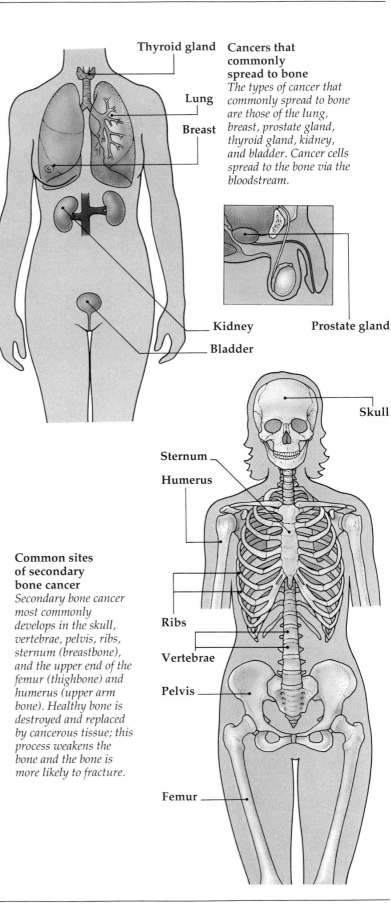

Cancers that commonly spread to bone
The types of cancer that commonly spread to bone are those of the lung, breast, prostate gland, thyroid gland, kidney, and bladder. Cancer cells spread to the bone via the bloodstream.

Thyroid gland

Lung

Breast

Kidney

Bladder

Prostate gland

Common sites of secondary bone cancer
Secondary bone cancer most commonly develops in the skull, vertebrae, pelvis, ribs, sternum (breastbone), and the upper end of the femur (thighbone) and humerus (upper arm bone). Healthy bone is destroyed and replaced by cancerous tissue; this process weakens the bone and the bone is more likely to fracture.

Skull

Sternum

Humerus

Ribs

Vertebrae

Pelvis

Femur

OSTEOMYELITIS

Osteomyelitis is an infection of the bone marrow and the surrounding bone. It is a disease that is more common in children, especially boys, and most often affects the long bones in the arms and legs and the vertebrae. Osteomyelitis is often caused by the bacterium *Staphylococcus aureus*, but can be caused by other organisms. The organism usually enters the bloodstream via a wound or infection of the skin and is carried to the bone. A diagnosis of osteomyelitis can be confirmed by blood tests and by X-rays and other imaging procedures.

THE STAGES OF OSTEOMYELITIS

Osteomyelitis most often affects the vertebrae and the long bones of the arms and legs. The disease exists in two forms – acute osteomyelitis and chronic osteomyelitis (see below). Chronic osteomyelitis most commonly develops if acute osteomyelitis is not treated or fails to respond to treatment. Chronic osteomyelitis can also occur after a fracture in which bone has pierced the skin.

Acute osteomyelitis
The disease begins with an infection (usually caused by bacteria) in a specific area of the bone. Acute osteomyelitis is treated with high doses of antibiotics over several weeks or months. With prompt treatment, acute osteomyelitis usually clears up completely.

Progression of osteomyelitis
If the infection persists, pus forms. Underlying bone dies and new bone forms. Symptoms include fever, chills, and bone pain. Treatment consists of surgery to clean out the dead bone area and pus, and long-term, high doses of an antibiotic.

Chronic osteomyelitis
New bone surrounds the area of infection, dead bone, and pus. The pus drains from the bone to the skin surface through channels, known as sinuses, in the bone. Treatment consists of antibiotics and surgical removal of the diseased or dead bone.

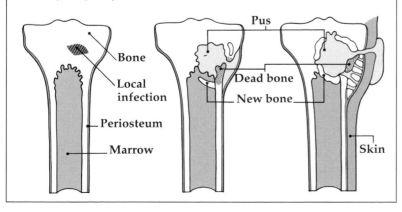

Bone
Local infection
Periosteum
Marrow
Pus
Dead bone
New bone
Skin

DEVELOPMENTAL PROBLEMS AFFECTING THE SKELETON

If a young child stands or walks differently from other children, his or her parents may become concerned. Most of these differences are nothing to worry about; they are a normal part of skeletal development and will go away as the child grows. However, some skeletal conditions require treatment.

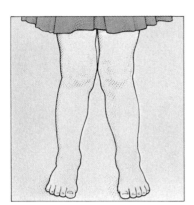

Knock-knees
Knock-knees are caused by an inward curving of the legs, so that when the child's knees touch, the ankles do not. This is a normal stage of development and requires no treatment unless the condition persists after age 10. Children with a persistent problem are usually treated by inserting heel wedges in their shoes to straighten the legs. In severe cases, an operation called an osteotomy may be needed to realign the leg bones.

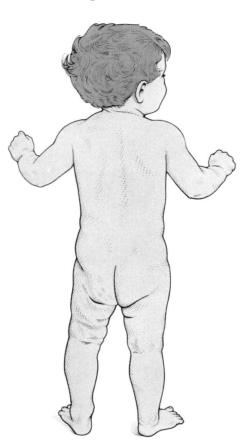

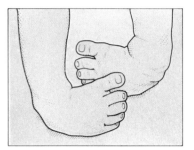

Clubfoot
Clubfoot is a deformity in which a baby is born with one or both feet bent downward and inward. All babies are checked for the disorder at birth. If your baby has this problem, your doctor will begin treatment as early as possible, including placing a cast on your baby's foot or feet. In some cases, this treatment corrects the problem. If the condition persists, surgery may be needed to cut tight ligaments and tendons and to realign the bones in the foot.

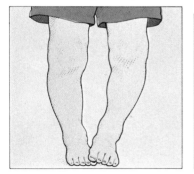

Bowlegs
In this condition, the child's legs curve outward, so that when the ankles touch (as above), the knees do not. Bowlegs are very common in children and are a normal stage of development. The outward curve usually straightens naturally. If your child has severely bowed legs or the condition lasts past age 6, you should consult your doctor.

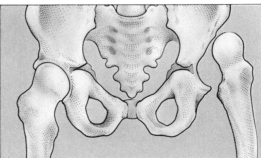

Congenital dislocation of the hip
Dislocation of the hip at birth (congenital dislocation) affects girls more often than boys. The ball of the femur (thighbone) lies outside the socket in the pelvis (lower illustration). All babies are checked for this condition at birth. Occasionally, the condition is not detected, as shown in the upper illustration; the extra skin folds below the left buttock indicate dislocation of the left hip. The condition runs in families, but its cause is not known. Correction by splinting is effective in the early stages.

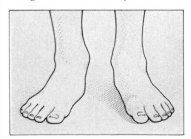

Flatfoot
Flatfoot is a condition in which the soles of the feet rest flat on the ground. All babies have flatfoot at birth; the arches begin to form naturally during the first 6 years of life. In some children, flatfoot persists and is usually painless and requires no treatment. Special exercises and arch supports are sometimes recommended. Surgery is rarely performed.

CASE HISTORY
A PAINFUL HEEL

JONATHAN, a car mechanic, had a sore left heel for about 4 weeks. The pain started after he jumped down into one of the grease pits in his garage to work on a customer's car. At first he thought he had a bad bruise and put an ice pack on his heel. But the soreness did not go away, and it was too painful to put his full weight on his left foot. Jonathan called his doctor.

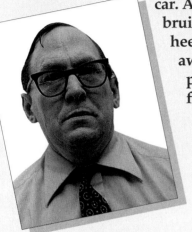

PERSONAL DETAILS
Name Jonathan Dietrich
Age 54
Occupation Car mechanic
Family Jonathan's parents are both healthy.

MEDICAL BACKGROUND
Jonathan broke his right ankle several years ago and the injury took 3 months to heal. Otherwise, he has had no serious health problems, although he occasionally suffers from minor bruises and muscle aches in the course of his work. Jonathan's weight is normal and he does not smoke.

THE CONSULTATION
Jonathan tells his doctor that he jumped down only about 4 feet, but that he landed awkwardly and jarred his left heel. Examination of his sore heel reveals an area of tenderness at the front of the heel pad, but no other abnormalities. There are no signs of tenderness or pain in his right heel.

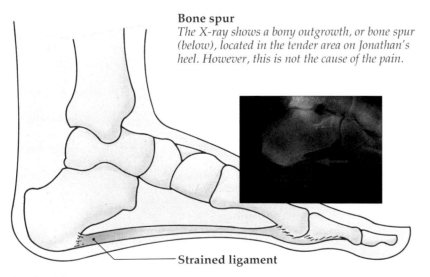

Bone spur
The X-ray shows a bony outgrowth, or bone spur (below), located in the tender area on Jonathan's heel. However, this is not the cause of the pain.

Strained ligament

Strained ligament
Jonathan's fall resulted in a strain of one of the ligaments that supports the arch of the foot at the point where it attaches to the heel bone.

THE DOCTOR'S IMPRESSION
The doctor thinks Jonathan's pain is the result of an injury to the soft tissues in his heel. To exclude the possibility of a fracture, he takes an X-ray of Jonathan's left foot. The X-ray shows no fracture, but the doctor notices an outgrowth of bone on the heel bone.

THE DIAGNOSIS
Jonathan's doctor tells him that he has a STRAINED LIGAMENT, which is causing the pain and tenderness in his left heel. The strain has caused inflammation of the ligament and surrounding tissues. The doctor also tells Jonathan that the bony outgrowth on the X-ray is a bone spur. The tender spot on Jonathan's heel coincides with the location of the bone spur and the strained ligament. The doctor explains that his pain is not being caused by the bone spur, and that bone spurs usually do not cause any symptoms. Jonathan is relieved because he thought he might need an operation to remove the bone spur.

THE TREATMENT
The doctor injects a mixture of an anesthetic and a corticosteroid drug into the tender area under Jonathan's heel. His pain subsides as the anesthetic takes effect, but the doctor tells him that the pain will return when it wears off. Jonathan's doctor prescribes an anti-inflammatory drug to be taken for 1 week, because the corticosteroid will take 2 or 3 days to relieve the inflammation of the ligament in his heel. The doctor also gives Jonathan a heel cushion to wear in his left shoe.

THE OUTCOME
Jonathan returns to see his doctor 1 week later. His heel is slightly tender and the doctor reassures him that within another 2 weeks the pain should be gone. Jonathan's doctor tells him to continue wearing the heel cushion for at least the next month.

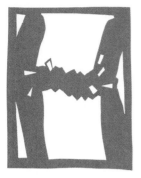

FRACTURES

THE "SETTING" OF BROKEN BONES is one of the oldest and most effective areas of medical care, with roots in early folk medicine traditions. Today's surgical techniques can repair fractures that in the past would have led to permanent disability. Research continues into ways to speed the healing of fractured bone.

The most common cause of a bone fracture is an injury. Fractures may also be caused by repeated stress on a bone, such as prolonged walking, marching, or even dancing. Minor injury or very slight stress, such as that caused by a vigorous cough or sneeze, can fracture a bone that already has been weakened by a disease such as osteoporosis (loss of protein and minerals from bone).

Fractures are usually divided into two categories – closed and open. In a closed fracture, the two ends of the broken bone remain under the skin. In an open (or compound) fracture, the end or ends of the bone project through the skin.

PATTERNS OF FRACTURE

Bones break in different ways, depending on the direction of the force applied to them. The pattern of the fracture helps your doctor determine the most effective treatment to heal the broken bone.

1. Transverse fracture
A direct blow to or an angular force on a bone that is held stable may cause a break straight across the bone (called a transverse fracture). The bone ends of a transverse fracture may remain aligned; the broken bone is immobilized in a cast to allow the fracture to heal.

2. Spiral fracture
A violent twisting movement can cause a spiral fracture of a long bone, such as the bones in the leg. A spiral fracture may be unstable, and the bone ends can damage blood vessels or nerves or break through the skin. Depending on the severity of the fracture, it may be treated with immobilization in a cast or with surgery.

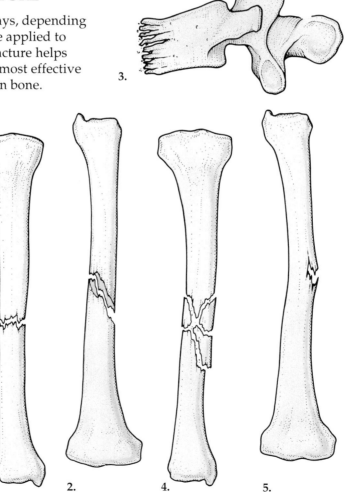

3. Crush fracture
Cancellous (spongy) bone, such as the bone in the vertebrae, can be crushed. This type of fracture can usually be treated with a brace. Some crush fractures can be hard to treat because of persistent pain and because the shape of the crushed vertebrae cannot be restored.

4. Comminuted fracture
In this type of fracture, which is most often caused by direct physical force, the bone is splintered into many fragments. This type of fracture may be difficult to treat because the bone fragments must be repositioned.

5. Greenstick fracture
If subjected to a strong force, the long bones in young children usually buckle and snap on one side. In most cases, this type of fracture is treated by immobilizing the bone in a cast.

TYPES OF FRACTURES

Bones tend to break at their weakest point. As we become older, our bones become weaker. A fall onto the outstretched hand in a young adult may fracture the scaphoid bone (a small bone in the wrist), while in an older person the fall may cause a fracture of the end of one of the forearm bones. An undisplaced fracture is one in which the fractured bone is cracked but the bone ends have not separated. In a displaced fracture, the two ends have separated.

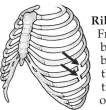

Rib fractures

Fractures of the ribs are common and can be very painful. They are usually caused by a fall or a strong blow to the side of the chest. Most rib fractures heal by themselves and require no treatment other than analgesic drugs (painkillers) and sometimes a rib belt for support. In some rib fractures, a fragment of bone pierces the lung, which requires treatment in the hospital. Severe pain and shortness of breath may indicate that a lung has been pierced and has collapsed. In severe chest injuries, the functioning of the lungs may be impaired and temporary mechanical ventilation may be needed.

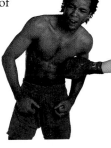

Fractured femur

A fracture of the neck of the femur (the part of the thighbone closest to the pelvis) most often occurs in older people whose bones have been weakened by osteoporosis. A person with a fracture of the neck of the femur experiences considerable pain and cannot walk. Surgery is almost always necessary; the bone ends are fitted back together or the head of the femur may be replaced, depending on the location of the fracture and the age of the person.

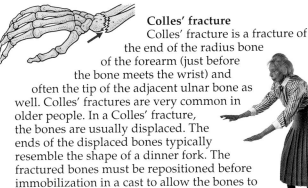

Ankle fractures

Ankle fractures often occur in young people as a result of sports injuries. When the ends of the broken bone are displaced, surgery is usually performed to bring the separated ends back together and keep them in place. After a fracture, swelling of the soft tissues around the ankle persists for some time after the fracture has healed. Although the swelling usually disappears over time, physical therapy and applying an elastic stocking or bandage to support the ankle may help reduce the swelling.

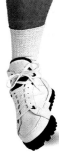

Colles' fracture

Colles' fracture is a fracture of the end of the radius bone of the forearm (just before the bone meets the wrist) and often the tip of the adjacent ulnar bone as well. Colles' fractures are very common in older people. In a Colles' fracture, the bones are usually displaced. The ends of the displaced bones typically resemble the shape of a dinner fork. The fractured bones must be repositioned before immobilization in a cast to allow the bones to heal properly.

Scaphoid fractures

The scaphoid bone of the wrist, which lies near the base of the thumb, can be injured by falling onto an outstretched hand. Fractures of the scaphoid bone are slow to heal and usually need to be immobilized for at least 3 months. In some cases, scaphoid fractures do not heal and an operation is required. Screws are used to hold the ends of the fractured bone tightly together or a small piece of bone is implanted to allow growth of bone and healing of the fracture.

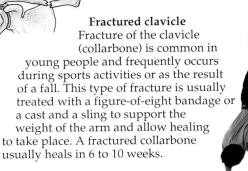

Fractured clavicle

Fracture of the clavicle (collarbone) is common in young people and frequently occurs during sports activities or as the result of a fall. This type of fracture is usually treated with a figure-of-eight bandage or a cast and a sling to support the weight of the arm and allow healing to take place. A fractured collarbone usually heals in 6 to 10 weeks.

SYMPTOMS AND DIAGNOSIS

Fractures usually cause swelling, tenderness, and an abnormal range of motion at the site of the fracture. In some cases, the bone is visibly deformed or the ends of the fractured bone project through the skin. The diagnosis of a fracture is confirmed by X-ray examination. X-rays also show the type of fracture and degree of displacement, if any, of the bone ends.

Fractured tibia
This color-enhanced X-ray shows a displaced fracture of the tibia (shinbone), one of the two bones in the lower part of the leg. The ends of the fractured bone have separated and moved out of alignment.

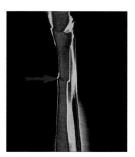

FRACTURE TREATMENT

Determination of the appropriate treatment for a fracture is based on several factors, including the type of fracture, the bone that is fractured, and your age.

If the ends of the fractured bone are not displaced, immobilization of the bone in a cast is often all that is required. If the ends of the fractured bone are separated, they must be manipulated back into their original position. This process is called reduction. Your doctor may be able to manipulate the bone ends back into the proper position without cutting open the tissue around the fracture. In some cases, surgery is required. Bone position is maintained by immobilization in a cast, by traction, or by pins, wires, screws, and plates.

External fixation
In the method of external fixation shown below, the position of the fractured bone is maintained by metal pins that are inserted through the skin into the bone and then attached to an external metal frame. External fixation requires minimal surgical intervention. It is especially useful because it helps prevent more injury to the severely injured muscle and skin around the area of the fractured bone.

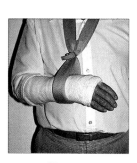

Immobilization in a cast
For many fractures, the bone is immobilized in a plaster cast (shown at left). Plastic casts are lighter than plaster and may permit better X-ray examination of a fracture while it is healing.

Traction
Traction is a means of maintaining the alignment of a fractured bone such as the femur (thighbone). The patient must remain in bed during the healing process, which may take several months.

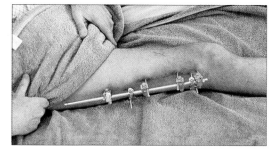

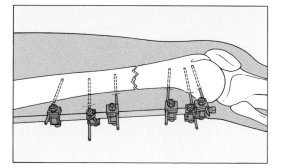

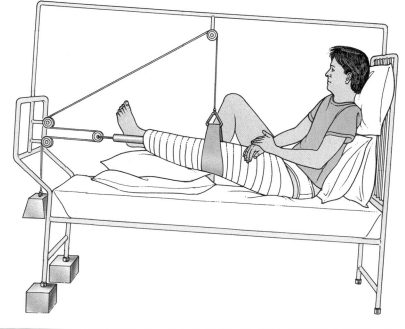

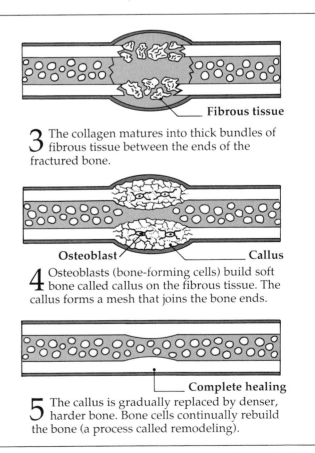

Internal fixation

Internal fixation of fractures became an effective technique after World War II when special metallic alloys were developed that were nonmagnetic and did not rust after being implanted into the body. Internal fixation allows a person to resume use of the injured limb more quickly, exercising adjacent joints and thereby preventing stiffness. Another advantage of being able to resume use of a limb soon after an injury is that the risk of muscle wasting and calcium loss from bone is decreased. However, internal fixation of a fracture does require surgery, and infection of the bone can occur, which complicates the healing process.

A fracture that has been fixed in place by plates and screws may take as long to heal as a fracture that is treated by immobilization in a cast. The reason for this is that the insertion of nails or another fixation device can disturb the blood supply to the bone, which delays healing.

Internal fixation
The illustration above shows four methods of internal fixation for immobilizing a fractured bone. From left to right they are: plate and screws, plates and compression screws, oblique transfixion screws, and a rod inserted into the hollow cavity (medullary canal) in the center of a long bone (see page 72). Internal fixation is usually used for fractures at the ends of the bones close to joints such as the hip, knee, ankle, elbow, wrist, and shoulder.

HOW BONES HEAL

A fractured bone starts to heal immediately. A fracture in a long bone of an adult normally takes about 6 to 12 weeks to heal. Fractures heal more quickly in children.

Blood clot

1 A blood clot forms between the ends of the fractured bone, sealing off any blood vessels that were damaged by the fracture.

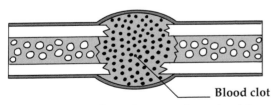

Fibroblast — **Shrinking clot** — **Collagen**

2 Fibroblasts form a fibrous protein called collagen between the ends of the bone. The clot is dissolved and removed by white blood cells.

Fibrous tissue

3 The collagen matures into thick bundles of fibrous tissue between the ends of the fractured bone.

Osteoblast — **Callus**

4 Osteoblasts (bone-forming cells) build soft bone called callus on the fibrous tissue. The callus forms a mesh that joins the bone ends.

Complete healing

5 The callus is gradually replaced by denser, harder bone. Bone cells continually rebuild the bone (a process called remodeling).

SURGICAL PROCEDURES
INTERNAL FIXATION OF A FRACTURED SHAFT OF FEMUR

FRACTURE OF THE SHAFT of the femur (thighbone) tends to occur as a result of a severe physical force, such as that involved in an automobile accident. In one type of treatment, called locked intramedullary nailing, a strong metal rod is inserted down the hollow cavity (medullary canal) in the center of the bone to hold a fractured bone together. The person can move his or her hip and knee immediately after the operation, which prevents joint stiffness, and can often put some weight on the injured leg soon after surgery. The person usually regains full use of the leg within 3 months after the operation.

Site of fracture

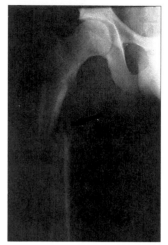

LOCKED INTRAMEDULLARY NAILING

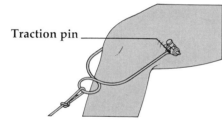

Traction pin

1 After administration of an anesthetic, the surgeon inserts a temporary traction pin into the end of the femur nearest the knee and applies traction to bring the ends of the fractured bone into alignment.

2 The surgeon makes an incision on the upper side of the buttock and makes a hole at the top end of the femur. He or she then passes a long, stiff wire (about the thickness of a wire coat hanger) down the medullary canal in the center of the broken bone, across the fracture and as far as the knee.

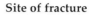
Guide wire   Incision   Femur

3 The surgeon enlarges the medullary canal with a special instrument and inserts a hollow, metal rod (the intramedullary rod) over the guide wire. The guide wire is then withdrawn.

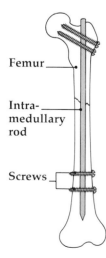

Femur

Intramedullary rod

Screws

4 To keep the bones stable, screws are inserted into the bone through the intramedullary rod. The surgeon makes another small incision at the lower end of the femur to insert screws into the other end of the rod. The incisions are then closed and the leg is elevated.

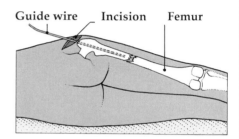

Intramedullary rod

Medullary canal

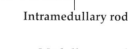
Guide wire

COMPLICATIONS OF FRACTURES

When a bone is fractured, the injury causes some degree of damage to surrounding tissues. Usually the damage is minor and repairs itself. In some cases, surgery is needed to repair a damaged nerve or artery or to release pressure around muscles. Infection of open fractures may occur and can be very serious (see OSTEOMYELITIS on page 65).

Sometimes a fracture reunites at the wrong angle. Surgery may be required to realign the bone. Bone healing may be delayed if the blood supply to the fractured bone is inadequate. If the bone does not heal, internal fixation may be required, often accompanied by bone grafting (implantation of bone from elsewhere in the body). The use of electrical stimulation to promote bone healing is being studied, but its treatment value remains unestablished.

Reflex sympathetic dystrophy (or Sudeck's atrophy) sometimes occurs after a fracture in an arm or leg bone. The condition is caused by spasm of the blood vessels in the injured area. After a fracture of the wrist, for example, the hand may become painful, stiff, and sweaty, with blotchy skin. This condition requires medical treatment.

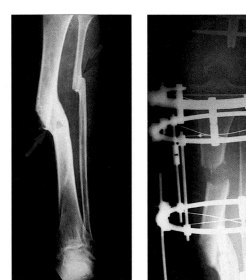

Treatment of improperly healed fractures
The X-ray on the far left shows fractures of the bones of the lower part of the right leg that have healed at the wrong angle (arrows). In the X-ray at left, an osteotomy (removal of bone) has been performed on each bone and the bones have been placed in a special device to correct the deformity caused by the improperly healed bones.

NEW BONE-GROWTH PROTEINS

Scientists have developed bone-growth proteins that may improve the treatment of fractures. The bone-growing compounds are made from collagen, a protein found in body tissues, combined with ceramic materials. They work by providing a framework upon which new bone can grow and by stimulating the body's natural process of bone growth. Scientists hope that the compounds will make it possible to repair severe fractures without a bone graft. Some scientists believe that it will someday be possible to heal serious fractures without surgery by injecting bone-growing compounds into the fractured area of the bone.

ASK YOUR DOCTOR
FRACTURES

Q Two years ago I broke both bones in my forearm. My doctor repaired the fractures using plates and screws. Do I need to have the plates and screws removed?

A If the plates and screws are not causing pain, swelling, or loss of motion, they do not need to be removed. There is a chance of infection or new fracture at the site of the holes left by the screws if plates and screws are removed.

Q My aunt broke her wrist, which was put in a cast. When the cast was removed, the wrist looked misshapen, although she is able to move it and it is not painful. Should she have the wrist reset, and is there an increased chance of arthritis in that wrist?

A If your aunt's wrist is working well, she doesn't need to have surgery to reset it. The risks of surgery and possible complications outweigh the benefit that may be achieved. Unless the fracture broke through into the wrist joint itself, there is minimal risk that arthritis will develop in that joint.

Q My 80-year-old mother has a broken hip. Her doctor tells me he must operate. Is surgery absolutely necessary at her age?

A The fracture could eventually heal by itself. However, despite her age, your mother's best chance of recovery is to have the surgery to repair the fracture and to get her back on her feet as soon as possible. It is dangerous for her to be immobilized in bed, because of the risk of pneumonia, bedsores, urinary tract infection, or other complications.

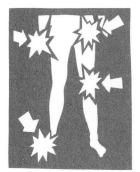

THE SPECTRUM OF JOINT DISEASE

T HE TERM "ARTHRITIS" describes a wide range of diseases that affect the joints. In general, all forms of arthritis are characterized by joint pain, swelling, and stiffness and a reduced range of motion in a joint. Arthritis can be broadly classified as osteoarthritis (or noninflammatory arthritis) and inflammatory arthritis.

Osteoarthritis, also called degenerative arthritis, is the most common form of arthritis. In weight-bearing joints, joint damage, malalignment, or instability can cause osteoarthritis. Obesity is another factor. Inflammatory arthritis is a general term for many arthritic diseases in which joints are inflamed.

THE EFFECTS OF ARTHRITIS

The National Institute of Arthritis and Musculoskeletal and Skin Diseases estimates that arthritis is the leading cause of disability in the US, with more than 37 million Americans affected by one or

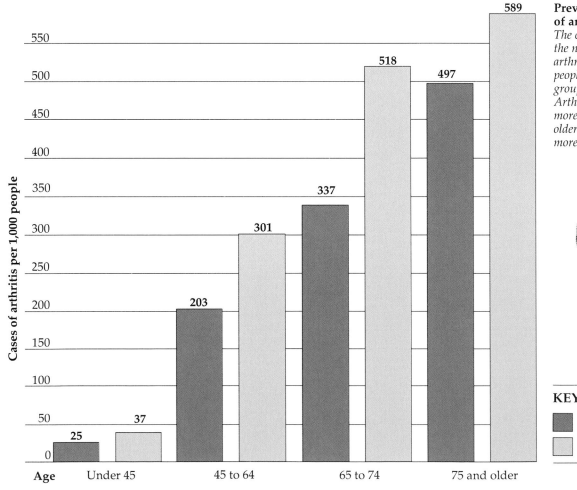

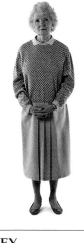

Prevalence of arthritis
The chart (left) shows the number of cases of arthritis per 1,000 people in different age groups in the US. Arthritis develops more commonly in older people and affects more women than men.

KEY

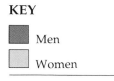
Men
Women

more of the arthritic diseases. Although the many forms of arthritis have symptoms in common, they differ in their causes and the damage they produce. In recent years, doctors have acquired a better understanding of arthritic diseases and, although the causes of some forms are still not known, many people are now being diagnosed and treated before the disease causes disability.

Defining arthritis

Arthritis can be classified by the number of joints affected – monarthritis involves one joint and polyarthritis affects several or many joints. The pattern of affected joints helps your doctor diagnose your condition. For example, symmetrical involvement of the small joints in both hands and feet may suggest rheumatoid arthritis; pain and stiffness in the lower part of the back may suggest ankylosing spondylitis (see pages 117 and 119).

Osteoarthritis
Osteoarthritis affects about 10 percent of the population. Almost everyone over the age of 60 has signs of osteoarthritis, but crippling disability caused by this condition is much less common. In osteoarthritis, the cartilage covering the bone ends becomes thin and begins to flake and crack. The underlying bone is exposed and eroded. Cysts develop in the exposed bone and outgrowths of bone, known as osteophytes, develop around the edges of the joint.

Inflammatory arthritis
In inflammatory arthritis, the synovial membrane, which lines the joint capsule, becomes thickened and swollen as a result of increased blood flow and infiltration with inflammatory cells. The bones become thin and often deformed. The most common form of inflammatory arthritis is rheumatoid arthritis, which affects and may cause disability in approximately 1 percent of the US population.

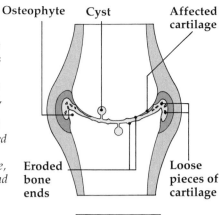
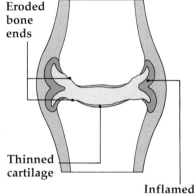

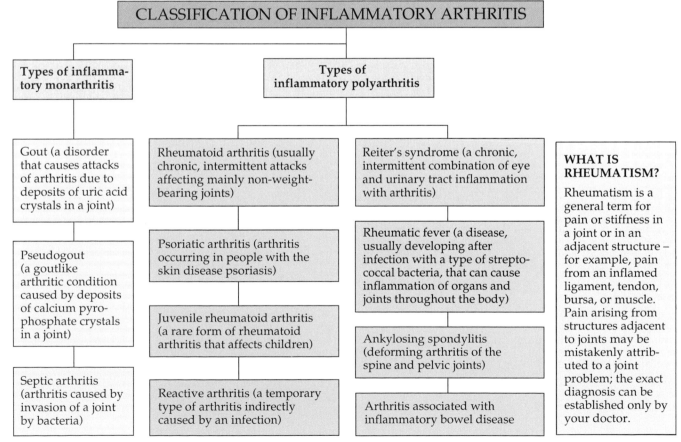

CLASSIFICATION OF INFLAMMATORY ARTHRITIS

Types of inflammatory monarthritis

Types of inflammatory polyarthritis

Gout (a disorder that causes attacks of arthritis due to deposits of uric acid crystals in a joint)

Pseudogout (a goutlike arthritic condition caused by deposits of calcium pyrophosphate crystals in a joint)

Septic arthritis (arthritis caused by invasion of a joint by bacteria)

Rheumatoid arthritis (usually chronic, intermittent attacks affecting mainly non-weight-bearing joints)

Psoriatic arthritis (arthritis occurring in people with the skin disease psoriasis)

Juvenile rheumatoid arthritis (a rare form of rheumatoid arthritis that affects children)

Reactive arthritis (a temporary type of arthritis indirectly caused by an infection)

Reiter's syndrome (a chronic, intermittent combination of eye and urinary tract inflammation with arthritis)

Rheumatic fever (a disease, usually developing after infection with a type of streptococcal bacteria, that can cause inflammation of organs and joints throughout the body)

Ankylosing spondylitis (deforming arthritis of the spine and pelvic joints)

Arthritis associated with inflammatory bowel disease

WHAT IS RHEUMATISM?
Rheumatism is a general term for pain or stiffness in a joint or in an adjacent structure – for example, pain from an inflamed ligament, tendon, bursa, or muscle. Pain arising from structures adjacent to joints may be mistakenly attributed to a joint problem; the exact diagnosis can be established only by your doctor.

MONITOR YOUR SYMPTOMS
PAINFUL OR SWOLLEN JOINTS

Pain and swelling in your joints can be distressing but may be simply a temporary symptom of an illness such as a viral infection. However, some types of joint pain are the result of a more serious condition and may require medical treatment.

Reactive arthritis (an inflammation of the joints that can accompany severe viral infections, such as hepatitis, measles, and mumps) may be responsible.

Action Call your doctor. He or she may prescribe medication. This type of joint pain usually goes away once the underlying infection has been treated.

BEGIN HERE

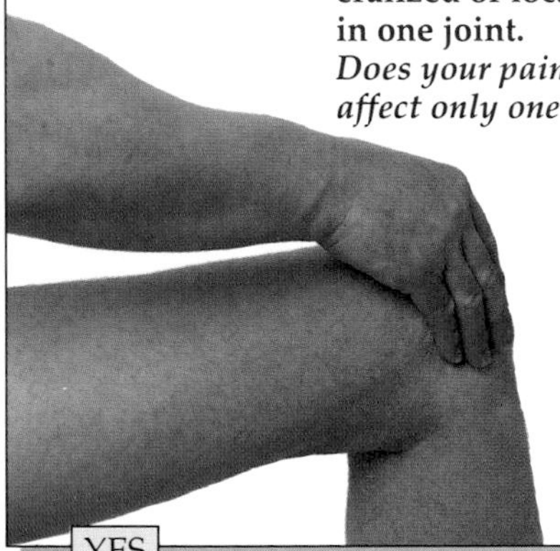

Joint pain can be generalized or localized in one joint.
Does your pain affect only one joint?

NO

Some infections can cause temporary joint pain.
Do you have a viral infection or have you recently had one?

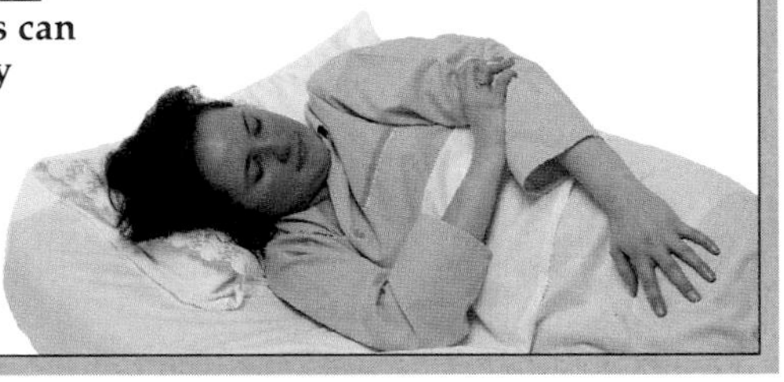

YES

NO

YES

Action Consult the chart
PAINFUL ARM OR LEG on page 42.

NO

YES

NO

You may have arthritis. The pattern of your symptoms helps your doctor diagnose the type of arthritis.
Does your pain tend to get worse toward the end of the day, especially if you have been active?

Joint pain may be sudden or may increase slowly over months or years.
Have you had increasing pain over a period of several years?

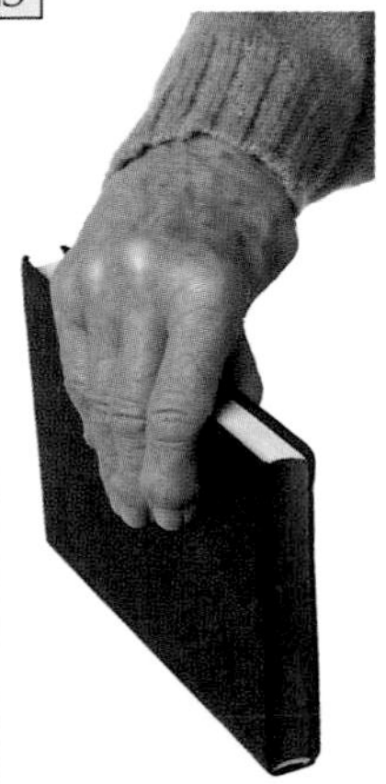

Rheumatoid arthritis (a long-term, inflammatory joint disease that can be disabling in its advanced stages) may be causing your problems. The disease most commonly affects the joints of the fingers, wrists, knees, and ankles. Rheumatoid arthritis can also produce symptoms such as fatigue or fever.

Action Call your doctor, who may arrange for you to have blood tests and X-rays. If the diagnosis of rheumatoid arthritis is confirmed, your doctor may prescribe medication. He or she may recommend that you see a physical therapist to learn exercises to keep your joints mobile.

YES

Osteoarthritis (degenerative arthritis), an arthritis associated with deterioration of the cartilage of the joint surface, is a possible cause of such pain, especially if you are over 50 and if you have regularly overused the joint.

Action See your doctor. He or she will examine you and may arrange for you to have a blood test and X-rays of the joints. If the diagnosis of osteoarthritis is confirmed, your doctor will prescribe medication and may refer you to a physical therapist.

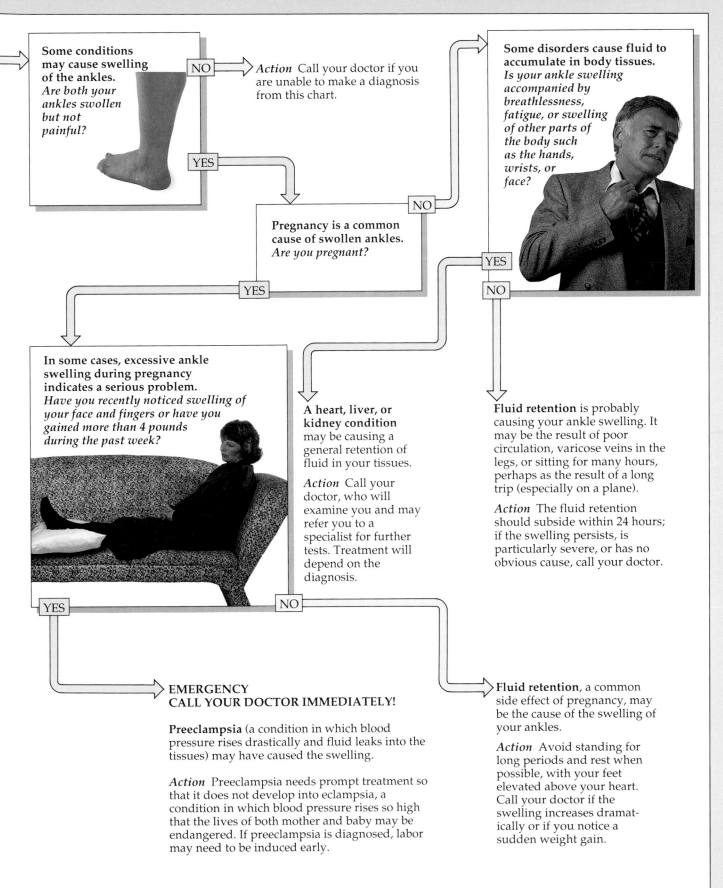

Some conditions may cause swelling of the ankles. *Are both your ankles swollen but not painful?*

NO → **Action** Call your doctor if you are unable to make a diagnosis from this chart.

YES ↓

Pregnancy is a common cause of swollen ankles. *Are you pregnant?*

NO →

Some disorders cause fluid to accumulate in body tissues. *Is your ankle swelling accompanied by breathlessness, fatigue, or swelling of other parts of the body such as the hands, wrists, or face?*

YES

NO

YES ↓

In some cases, excessive ankle swelling during pregnancy indicates a serious problem. *Have you recently noticed swelling of your face and fingers or have you gained more than 4 pounds during the past week?*

A heart, liver, or kidney condition may be causing a general retention of fluid in your tissues.

Action Call your doctor, who will examine you and may refer you to a specialist for further tests. Treatment will depend on the diagnosis.

Fluid retention is probably causing your ankle swelling. It may be the result of poor circulation, varicose veins in the legs, or sitting for many hours, perhaps as the result of a long trip (especially on a plane).

Action The fluid retention should subside within 24 hours; if the swelling persists, is particularly severe, or has no obvious cause, call your doctor.

YES

NO

EMERGENCY CALL YOUR DOCTOR IMMEDIATELY!

Preeclampsia (a condition in which blood pressure rises drastically and fluid leaks into the tissues) may have caused the swelling.

Action Preeclampsia needs prompt treatment so that it does not develop into eclampsia, a condition in which blood pressure rises so high that the lives of both mother and baby may be endangered. If preeclampsia is diagnosed, labor may need to be induced early.

Fluid retention, a common side effect of pregnancy, may be the cause of the swelling of your ankles.

Action Avoid standing for long periods and rest when possible, with your feet elevated above your heart. Call your doctor if the swelling increases dramatically or if you notice a sudden weight gain.

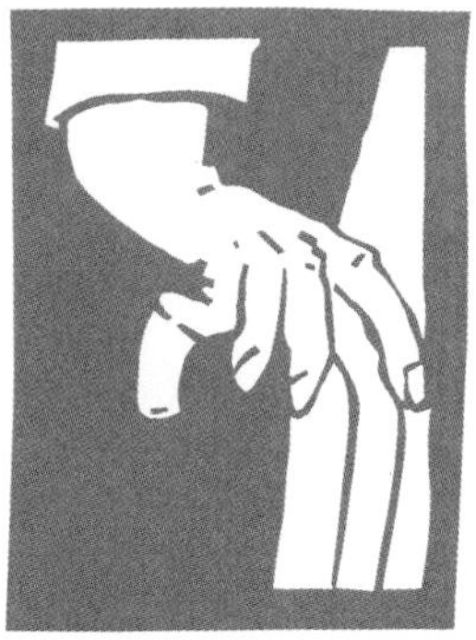

OSTEOARTHRITIS

O STEOARTHRITIS is a common joint disease and is the main cause of disability among older people. About 100,000 people in the US suffer from severe osteoarthritis. Osteoarthritis is sometimes called degenerative arthritis. In an affected joint, the cartilage on the ends of the bones progressively wears away.

Osteoarthritis may occur without apparent cause but is often the result of several poorly understood processes or disorders affecting the joints. It can occur as a result of repeated injury to a joint. Osteoarthritis may develop in several joints or may affect only one joint.

Joints most often affected by osteoarthritis
Joints that are commonly affected by osteoarthritis are those of the spine, the hands, the hips, the knees, and the feet.

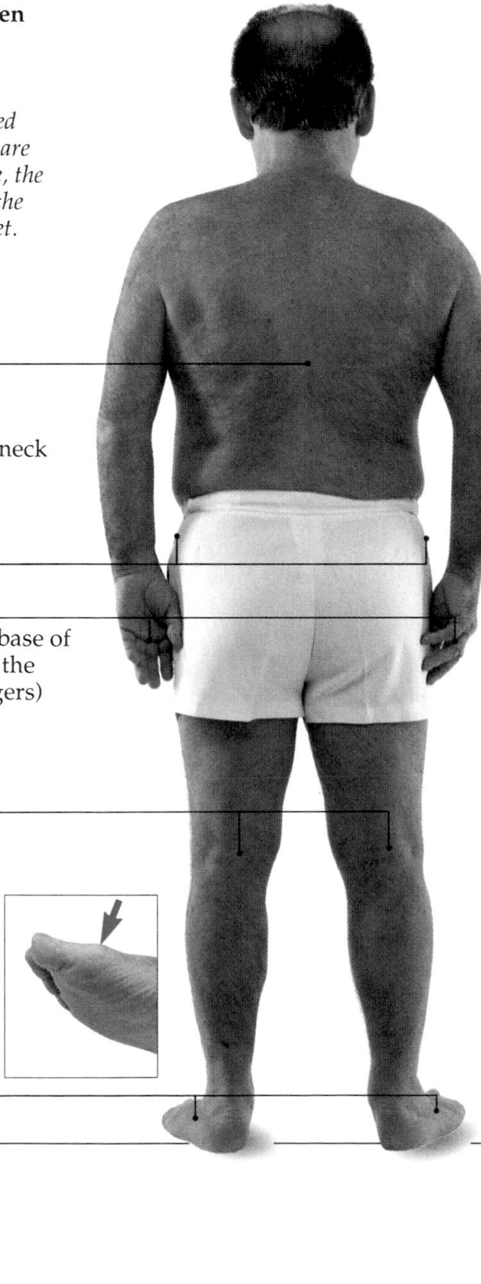

Spine
(especially the neck and lower part of the back)

Hips

Hands
(especially the base of the thumb and the ends of the fingers)

Knees

Feet
(mainly the joint at the base of the big toe)

WHO IS AFFECTED?

Osteoarthritis most commonly affects middle-aged and older people; the average age of onset of the disease is around 55. Results of studies using X-rays suggest that about 10 percent of all adults (and nearly everyone over age 60) has some degree of osteoarthritis, whether or not they experience symptoms. Osteoarthritis occurs more frequently in women than in men (by a ratio of about three to one) and occurs particularly frequently in white women.

TYPES AND CAUSES OF OSTEOARTHRITIS

Osteoarthritis that does not have an obvious cause is called primary osteoarthritis. If several of your joints are affected (see illustration at left), your doctor may use the term "generalized osteoarthritis" to describe your condition. Primary osteoarthritis usually affects middle-aged and older people.

Secondary osteoarthritis develops when cartilage covering the bone surfaces in a joint has been damaged – for example, by infection or by a fracture into the joint. Secondary osteoarthritis can occur at any age after mature bone growth has been reached. Children's joints can recover to some extent from an injury because of their bone-growth potential – an ability that is lost with age.

As our understanding of osteoarthritis improves, the division of osteoarthritis into primary and secondary forms is becoming less clear-cut. We now know that osteoarthritis may result from a combination of factors. These factors may include an injury, obesity, or a metabolic disorder such as acromegaly (enlargement of bones caused by excess secretion of growth hormone). However, your doctor can often determine one main causative factor. Some forms of osteoarthritis also seem to be inherited. Recently, it has been found that abnormal cartilage proteins that are present in some people may be a factor in allowing general breakdown of cartilage.

SYMPTOMS

Osteoarthritis can cause joint stiffness, pain, and restriction of movement of the affected joint. The joints may make crackling sounds during movement. Pain worsens toward the end of the day. People with osteoarthritis often describe the pain as a deep, aching sensation. Stiffness occurs mainly after periods of inactivity – the joints "freeze up" or "lock" and it can take several minutes of activity to "loosen" the joints again.

WHAT HAPPENS TO A JOINT AFFECTED BY OSTEOARTHRITIS?

The development of osteoarthritis follows a characteristic pattern.

1 Normal articular cartilage – the weight-bearing surface of the joint – is smooth and slippery, allowing low-friction movement of the joint.

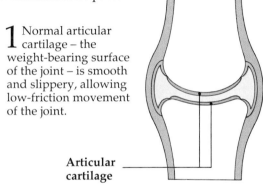

Articular cartilage

2 In the early stages of osteoarthritis, the articular cartilage begins to break down. The cartilage surfaces become rough and gradually become thinner as they move against each other. Small pieces of articular cartilage break off and may irritate the synovial membrane lining the inside of the joint capsule and cause excess joint fluid to form. The membrane becomes inflamed, painful, and thickened. The range of movement of the joint may be limited.

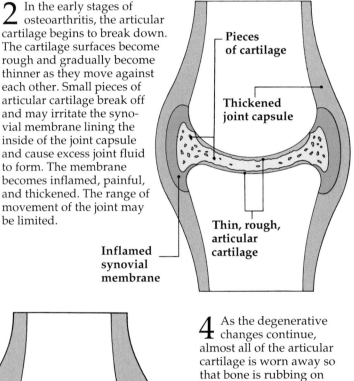

Pieces of cartilage

Thickened joint capsule

Thin, rough, articular cartilage

Inflamed synovial membrane

3 At this stage, the joint often forms outgrowths of articular cartilage and bone (called osteophytes) around its edges, giving the joint a knobby, swollen appearance.

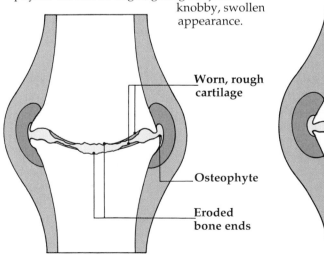

Worn, rough cartilage

Osteophyte

Eroded bone ends

4 As the degenerative changes continue, almost all of the articular cartilage is worn away so that bone is rubbing on bone, and the pain becomes more severe. Eventually, movement may be substantially limited.

Bone rubbing on bone

DIAGNOSING OSTEOARTHRITIS

Your doctor can make a diagnosis of osteoarthritis based on your symptoms, your history of joint problems, and a physical examination. The physical signs of osteoarthritis include tenderness of the affected joint, bony swellings (called osteophytes), pain and crackling noises (called crepitus) when the joint is moved, mild signs of inflammation (such as swelling, redness, and tenderness), and loss of the joint's full normal range of movement. X-rays of the joint usually confirm the diagnosis.

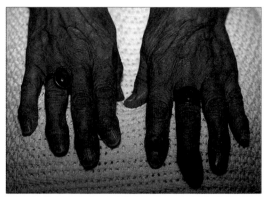

Bony swellings
Osteoarthritis may cause the finger joints to become enlarged and distorted by osteophytes (bony swellings), as shown above. Hands that have been affected by osteoarthritis may appear deformed, but often there is little disability.

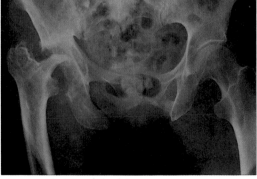

Osteoarthritis of the hip
This X-ray shows the pelvis of a person with osteoarthritis. The bones in the right hip (at left side of image) have been almost completely destroyed by osteoarthritis and the hip joint may need to be replaced (see page 82). The bones in the left hip (at right side of image) show less severe degeneration.

LIVING WITH OSTEOARTHRITIS

Although there is no cure for osteoarthritis, there are many things you can do to help relieve or reduce your symptoms and make it easier to live with the condition.

Slowing progression and preventing flare-ups
In many cases, joints are only mildly affected by osteoarthritis and flare-ups occur only occasionally over many years. You should try to reduce stresses and strains on your joints. Placing strain on a joint is likely to provoke a flare-up of painful symptoms. Being overweight also increases the rate at which the damaged cartilage in a joint wears away.

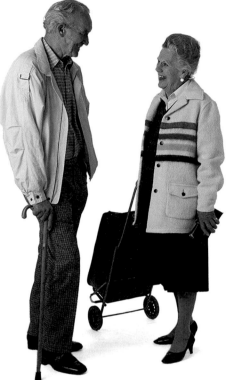

Reducing strain on your joints
The most common cause of strain on the joints is being overweight. Losing weight can help relieve the strain. You can also reduce strain on your joints by not carrying heavy objects and by walking with a cane.

Your state of mind
Talk to your doctor if you are feeling anxious about your condition. Depression and anxiety can lower your threshold for pain. In some people, treatment for depression is more useful than increasing the dosage of painkilling medication.

Your interests
Adjusting to a lower level of activity can be frustrating. You may have to develop new hobbies and physical activities. High-repetition, low-load exercises are better for you than high-impact activities. For example, walking is better than jogging.

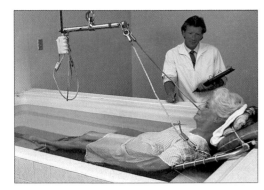

Hydrotherapy
Hydrotherapy, in which you soak in a tub of warm water and perform exercises under the guidance of a health professional, may help relieve your symptoms temporarily.

Heat treatment
Warmth helps alleviate symptoms. Keep your home well-heated in the winter and wear warm clothing. Massaging a joint or applying gentle heat with a heating pad, heat lamp, or hot water bottle can also help. The soothing comfort of the warm water of a bath, shower, whirlpool, or heated pool relieves painful joints and eases stiffness. Your doctor may recommend exercises to increase your flexibility and mobility.

Staying active
Regular, moderate exercise maintains the flexibility of your joints. To avoid problems caused by too much or too little activity, exercise moderately and often. For example, take short rests during your housework or gardening. Avoid sitting in one place for too long; get up, stretch your joints, and move about from time to time. Your doctor may recommend an exercise program supervised by a health professional.

Gentle exercise
Swimming is a good form of exercise that does not strain your joints. It is particularly appropriate if you have hip and knee problems. Modified aerobic exercise programs for people with arthritis are available in many communities. Participating in supervised programs approved by your doctor can improve function and decrease pain.

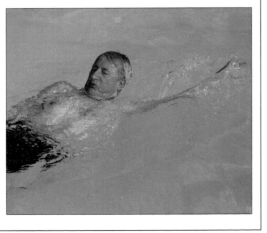

Drug treatment
Your doctor will probably prescribe a nonsteroidal anti-inflammatory drug (NSAID). The pain and discomfort of osteoarthritis are best relieved by taking a consistent dose of an NSAID such as aspirin at the lowest dose that provides maximum relief. If severe inflammation occurs during a flare-up of osteoarthritis, it can be relieved with an injection of a corticosteroid drug into the joint. However, injections should be limited to three or four into the same joint per year.

ASK YOUR DOCTOR
OSTEOARTHRITIS

Q I have severe osteoarthritis in my knee. My doctor has recommended that I have surgery to replace the knee joint. I have heard that the results of knee replacements are not as good as those of hip replacements. Is this true?

A The results of knee joint replacements being done today are nearly as good as those of hip joint replacements. If the disability and pain caused by the osteoarthritis in your knee are severe, a knee replacement is justified.

Q Are there any special diets that prevent osteoarthritis or slow the progression of the condition?

A No. Although some people believe that a particular diet has helped, there is no scientific evidence that any kind of diet influences the development or progression of osteoarthritis. If you are overweight, losing weight will relieve symptoms of osteoarthritis. Talk to your doctor about the type of diet that would be best for you.

Q My artificial hip joint was functioning well until a few months ago when I had an infected tooth removed. I now have a great deal of pain and stiffness in my hip. Should I see my doctor about this?

A You should see your doctor immediately. The infection from the tooth may have entered your bloodstream and moved into your hip. Always tell any doctor or dentist who treats you that you have an artificial hip joint. Depending on the procedures that are performed, he or she may prescribe antibiotics to protect against infection.

SURGICAL PROCEDURES
HIP JOINT REPLACEMENT

HIP JOINT replacement operations have relieved pain and restored mobility in many people with arthritis. In this operation, both the pelvic socket and the head of the femur (thighbone), which fits into the socket, are replaced. The joint components have traditionally been attached to the normal bone with an acrylic cement. However, loosening can occur over time. In an attempt to overcome this problem, cementless prostheses are being developed into which the person's own bone can grow.

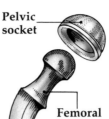

Pelvic socket

Femoral component

Artificial hip joint
The artificial hip joint (shown at left) consists of two parts. The pelvic socket is usually made of a strong plastic. It is often strengthened by a coating of metal. The femoral component is made of metal and consists of the head and neck and a long stem that fits down into the canal inside the femur.

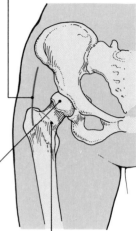

Skin incision

Head of femur

Bone incision

1 After cleaning the skin with an antiseptic, the surgeon makes an incision and exposes the hip joint. He or she cuts selected ligaments and muscles and removes the affected head of the femur by cutting across the neck of the bone.

Head of femur

2 The surgeon cleans out the area in the pelvis using an instrument called a reamer and puts the replacement socket in position. An acrylic cement can be used to hold the component in place, or the component may be fitted tightly into the bone so that it does not move.

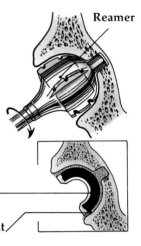

Reamer

New socket in position

Cement

3 The surgeon cleans out the hollow canal in the femur and implants the femoral component. As with the socket component, acrylic cement may be used, or the component may be fitted tightly in place.

4 The surgeon fits the head of the femoral component into the pelvic socket and closes the incision.

5 After 5 to 10 days, the patient may be discharged from the hospital. Initially, a walker and then a cane may be helpful for walking. The person is given exercises to do that help strengthen the muscles around the hip. For the first 12 weeks, there is a risk that the hip joint components may dislocate. To reduce the risks, most surgeons recommend that the person sleep with a pillow between his or her legs.

After the replacement surgery
This X-ray shows the hip joint components in position.

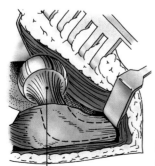

Femoral component

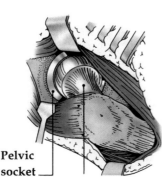

Pelvic socket

Femoral component

SURGERY FOR OSTEOARTHRITIS

Surgical treatment of arthritis is now extremely effective. Joint replacement (called arthroplasty) has been successfully performed on thousands of people. Arthroplasty has been used on the hips, knees, and ankles, as well as the small joints of the hands, wrists, and toes. Arthrodesis (fusion of the bones in a joint) immobilizes the joint and is used only in situations where it has been proved to produce a good long-term result – such as for osteoarthritis of the big toe. Arthrodesis of the ankle may be performed if pain is very severe. Osteotomy (cutting of a bone adjacent to a joint) may be done for young people who have osteoarthritis of the hip or knee. It causes stresses on the affected joint to be redistributed, enabling the arthritic hip or knee to continue functioning for a longer period of time.

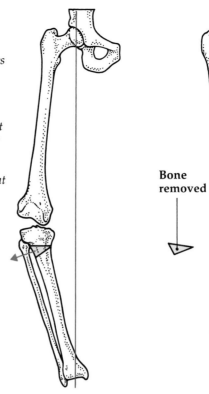

Osteotomy of the knee
Often, one of the bones of the knee joint becomes worn on one side while the other side remains normal; this moves the joint out of alignment. A wedge from the intact side of the affected bone is removed. The bone heals at a new angle, correcting the alignment of the joint.

Bone removed

Malaligned joint   **Realigned joint**

Knee joint prosthesis

Hip joint prosthesis

New life for worn-out joints
Joint replacements of the hip and knee have been very successful. Varying degrees of success have been achieved with replacement of shoulder, elbow, wrist, ankle, and even finger joints, and improvements continue to be made. Some types of knee and hip joint prostheses are shown here.

Arthrodesis of the big toe
The weight-bearing surfaces of the joint are removed. Ends of bones are held together with an internal fixation device – in this case, a type of screw – and with plaster. The bones unite as they heal and the joint is immovable.

Fixation device

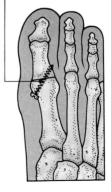

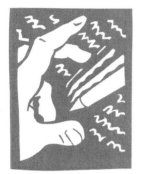

RHEUMATOID ARTHRITIS

RHEUMATOID ARTHRITIS is a serious type of joint disease. The condition takes various forms. In all cases, rheumatoid arthritis causes inflammation, pain, and stiffness in the affected joints. Rheumatoid arthritis can appear without warning and, in some cases, it disappears just as suddenly. In persistent cases, the joints are weakened and eventually become deformed so that function is substantially or completely impaired.

Rheumatoid arthritis is the most common inflammatory joint disease. Some forms of the disease occur only during childhood. The symptoms and severity of the disease vary from person to person. People who have mild forms of the disease are often described as having "possible" or "probable" rheumatoid arthritis, as opposed to the definite or classic form. Rheumatoid arthritis mainly affects the joints but in severe cases may involve other tissues.

HOW RHEUMATOID ARTHRITIS AFFECTS A JOINT

When a joint is affected by rheumatoid arthritis, the synovial membrane that lines the joint becomes inflamed, causing heat, swelling, and pain around the joint. If the disease persists, the inflammation spreads across the surface of the joint, causing the cartilage covering the ends of the bones to become irregular and thinner and eventually eroded. The inflammation also spreads to the joint capsule and the ligaments and tendons surrounding the joint, causing more pain and stiffness.

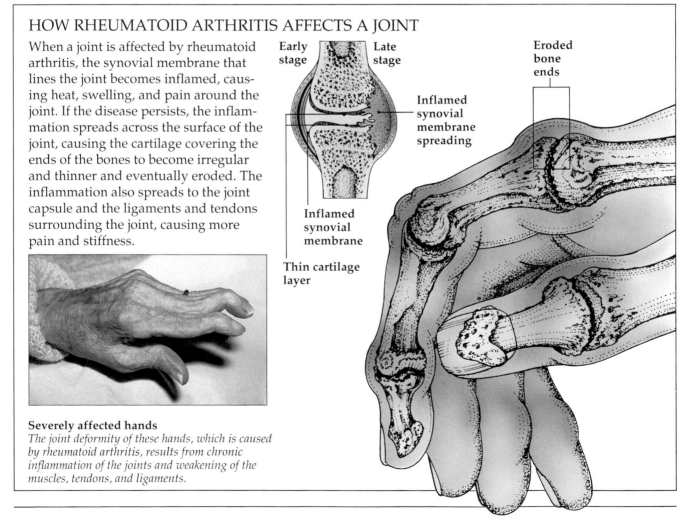

Early stage **Late stage**

Eroded bone ends

Inflamed synovial membrane spreading

Inflamed synovial membrane

Thin cartilage layer

Severely affected hands
The joint deformity of these hands, which is caused by rheumatoid arthritis, results from chronic inflammation of the joints and weakening of the muscles, tendons, and ligaments.

WHAT CAUSES RHEUMATOID ARTHRITIS?

We do not know the cause of rheumatoid arthritis, although the process of development of the disease is well understood. Some people inherit genetic characteristics that can increase the likelihood that the disease will develop. In some susceptible people there may be some kind of "trigger" incident, such as an infection, after which the disease becomes evident. Once the first episode of inflammation begins, the body's immune system seems to attack the joint tissues.

Incidence

Severe rheumatoid arthritis appears to be more common in northern Europe than elsewhere in the world, but there is no obvious pattern of distribution worldwide. In the US about one in 100 people has rheumatoid arthritis. The disease develops between ages 35 and 50 in the majority of affected people. Rheumatoid arthritis affects three times more women than men. Approximately one in 1,000 children is affected by a juvenile form of the disease (see page 96).

Symptoms

Most people with rheumatoid arthritis first notice tiredness and a feeling of being sick, followed by pain and stiffness in one or more joints. The joints that are usually affected first are those in the fingers, wrists, feet, or knees. Only one joint may be affected at first (monarticular rheumatoid arthritis) or problems with several joints may be noticed simultaneously (polyarticular rheumatoid arthritis). The affected joints are swollen, painful, warm, red, and stiff; the stiffness is most noticeable in the morning. Structures around the joints may become inflamed, resulting in weakness of the ligaments, tendons, and muscles.

As the disease progresses, more joints may become painful and swollen. The affected joints may become stiff, less

DIAGNOSING RHEUMATOID ARTHRITIS

The initial diagnosis of rheumatoid arthritis is usually based on the nature and history of the person's symptoms. The diagnosis is confirmed by taking X-rays of affected joints, such as those of the foot (below left) and knee (below right). Specific blood tests are also done, including tests for an antibody called rheumatoid factor. In some cases, synovial fluid is removed from inside an affected joint and analyzed to see if the white blood cell count is increased (an indication of an inflammatory condition), or a needle biopsy sample of synovial tissue is examined for the characteristics of rheumatoid arthritis.

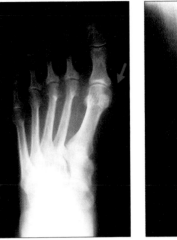 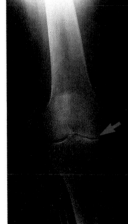

Rheumatoid foot
This X-ray of a left foot affected by rheumatoid arthritis shows bone erosion of the joint at the base of the big toe (arrow) and of the first joints of the other toes.

Rheumatoid knee
This X-ray of a right knee affected by rheumatoid arthritis shows narrowing of the joint space (arrow). The bone is also thinner than normal as a result of loss of minerals from the bone.

functional, and deformed. Between 10 and 20 percent of people with symptoms of rheumatoid arthritis recover completely within a few years of onset of the disease. In some people (5 to 10 percent), the pain and deformity develop rapidly and cause severe disability. In about 70 to 80 percent of people, the disease progresses slowly, with periodic flare-ups of symptoms alternating with periods when the symptoms almost disappear, leaving the person to cope with any residual joint deformities. In people with chronic rheumatoid arthritis, associated problems may develop in the nerves, eyes, lungs, skin, and blood vessels.

ASK YOUR DOCTOR
RHEUMATOID ARTHRITIS

Q **What is the difference between seropositive and seronegative rheumatoid arthritis?**

A About 80 percent of people with rheumatoid arthritis have an antibody called rheumatoid factor in their blood. If rheumatoid factor is present, the condition is known as seropositive rheumatoid arthritis; if it is not present (yet the person has other features of rheumatoid arthritis), the condition is known as seronegative. Seropositive arthritis is usually more severe than seronegative.

Q **My mother has severe rheumatoid arthritis. Is there a genetic susceptibility to the condition?**

A No single gene is responsible for causing rheumatoid arthritis. However, about 30 to 50 percent of people with rheumatoid arthritis have certain genetically determined markers in their body tissues, called HLAs (human leukocyte antigens), that are not usually found in the general population. These antigens play an important role in affecting the body's immune system, which attacks the joints once rheumatoid arthritis develops.

Q **What do doctors mean when they talk about a condition called intermittent arthritis?**

A Many people with rheumatoid arthritis have symptoms all of the time. About 25 percent have intermittent arthritis, which means that they have periods of arthritis that last many months, followed by remissions that last for a few months to many years.

TREATING RHEUMATOID ARTHRITIS

No cure currently exists for rheumatoid arthritis. Treatment is directed at relieving the symptoms, preventing joint deformity, and maintaining the mobility and stability of the joint. Drug therapy is used to relieve pain and inflammation and also to cause remission of the disease. Exercise is recommended to keep the joints mobile and stable and to maintain or improve physical fitness. Flare-ups of symptoms are treated with rest. Surgery may be needed to release tendons that have contracted around affected joints, to remove the inflamed synovial membrane (see below), and to remove damaged articular cartilage. Occasionally, joint deformity and immobility associated with pain can be treated with joint replacement surgery.

SYNOVECTOMY

If inflammation of the synovial membrane that lines a joint is persistent and disabling, a person with severe rheumatoid arthritis may be advised to have a synovectomy – surgical removal of the synovial membrane. This operation is performed only after drug therapy has been unsuccessful. Synovectomy can improve joint symptoms and delay progression of the disease for years but it cannot cure the underlying condition. Surgery such as joint replacement may be required later.

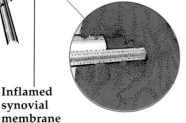

Power shaver

The operation
The inflamed synovial membrane may be removed using an arthroscope and a power shaver inserted through small incisions over the joint (the knee joint is shown here). In other cases, the synovial membrane is exposed with one large incision and then cut away.

Arthroscope

Inflamed synovial membrane

CASE HISTORY
STIFF, SWOLLEN FINGERS

Elaine Haverland, a jeweler, had noticed increasing stiffness, swelling, and pain in her fingers during the past few weeks. Some days she found it hard to hold the setting and cutting instruments she used at work, especially in the mornings. She decided to make an appointment to see her doctor.

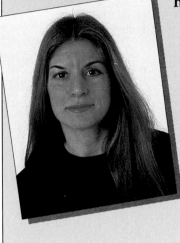

PERSONAL DETAILS
Name Elaine Haverland
Age 40
Occupation Jeweler
Family Both parents are well.

MEDICAL BACKGROUND
Elaine has been in fairly good health. About 3 months ago she had a severe case of bronchitis (inflammation of the air passages of the lungs). Her doctor prescribed antibiotics and her condition improved over 3 weeks. However, Elaine then noticed stiffness, swelling, and pain in her hands that usually lasted for 2 or 3 hours after she woke up.

THE CONSULTATION
Elaine describes the stiffness, swelling, and pain she has been having in her fingers. Elaine's doctor asks her if she has had a fever or has lost weight recently. She says she hasn't lost weight and hasn't felt like she has had a fever, but that she has been feeling very tired and that her muscles ache. Her doctor examines her hands and notices that she has swelling in the finger joints nearest her palms. The outer joints appear normal. Elaine's doctor then examines her other joints but finds they have not been affected.

FURTHER INVESTIGATION
Elaine's doctor takes a blood sample and sends it to the laboratory for tests. The laboratory report indicates that the test results for rheumatoid factor (an antibody produced by the body's immune system that is present in rheumatoid arthritis) are positive. An X-ray shows no signs of destructive changes in Elaine's finger joints.

THE DIAGNOSIS
Elaine's doctor tells her that the results of the physical examination and blood tests strongly suggest that she has RHEUMATOID ARTHRITIS. Her doctor explains that, although there is no cure for the disease, treatment can relieve symptoms and maintain the function of her affected joints.

THE TREATMENT
Elaine's doctor prescribes aspirin (a nonsteroidal anti-inflammatory drug) four times a day to relieve her symptoms and tells her to rest for an hour each day. Her doctor also gives her a program of exercises to keep her fingers mobile. If her symptoms persist despite treatment and there are signs of progression of the disease, Elaine's doctor says he may prescribe an antirheumatic drug, which might stop or slow the progression of the disease.

THE OUTCOME
Elaine's symptoms are relieved rapidly with the treatment. After 3 years it appears that the condition is no longer active. Elaine's doctor tells her that she is probably one of the fortunate 10 to 20 percent who have a complete remission of symptoms.

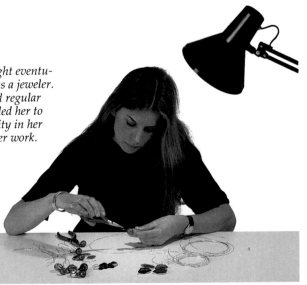

Manual dexterity
Elaine thought that she might eventually have to stop her work as a jeweler. Treatment with aspirin and regular exercise of her fingers enabled her to minimize the loss of dexterity in her hands and continue with her work.

LIVING WITH RHEUMATOID ARTHRITIS

Severe rheumatoid arthritis is a progressively disabling condition, but there are many aids available to help people with the disease perform everyday tasks safely and easily. These techniques and devices can help you remain independent. By using some of these aids you will also be exercising your muscles and joints, which will help keep them mobile.

Comfortable chair
It is very important to use a chair that you find comfortable and that also gives you support. Choose one with a firm back and try not to slouch. Arm rests provide support for your hands and arms and make it easier for you to get up from the chair.

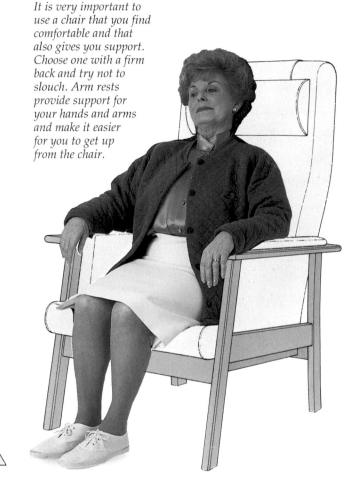

Book rest
A book rest alleviates the discomfort of having to hold a book in position for reading and allows you to rest your hands while you read.

Pen or pencil holder
If you have a weak grip, don't strain your fingers by using a thin pen or pencil. Give yourself a larger circumference to grasp by wrapping your pen or pencil with a pad of foam rubber.

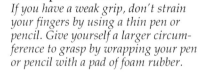

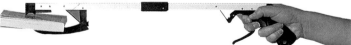

Tongs
Tongs like these will help you get a firm grip on objects that are out of your reach. When you are sitting down you can use the tongs to grasp objects and bring them to you without having to get up.

Kitchen work
Use a high stool at a kitchen counter to avoid strain on your joints. Be sure that you use a stool that you can get on to and down from easily. Specially adapted knives and other kitchen tools are available that are easy to grip.

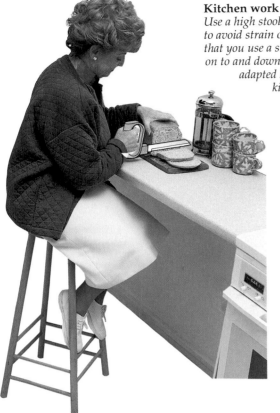

Special techniques
Use your forearms to support a tray as you carry it; this is easier than using your fingers and hands to grip the sides of the tray.

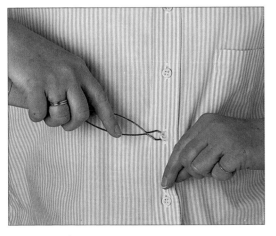

Tidying up
Long-handled tools for the house and garden help you do chores without bending.

Buttonhook
Fastening a button can be a difficult task for people with rheumatoid arthritis. A buttonhook can be inserted through the buttonhole and used to grip the button and pull it through.

Safety in the bath
A seat can be fitted in your bathtub so that you can get in and out easily. If you prefer to take showers, you can have a seat put in your shower. Handrails provide support getting in and out of the bathtub or shower.

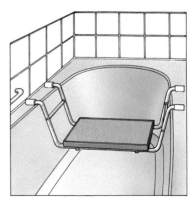

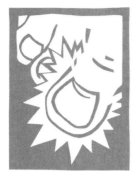

LESS COMMON FORMS OF ARTHRITIS

SEVERAL HUNDRED different diseases that attack the joints can be grouped under the heading of arthritis. This section discusses the causes, symptoms, and treatment of some forms of arthritis that, although not nearly as common as osteoarthritis or rheumatoid arthritis, cause disability in many people.

The causes of the less common types of arthritis are metabolic and biochemical abnormalities, infections, and disorders of the body's immune system.

ARTHRITIS CAUSED BY GOUT

Gout is a metabolic disorder that causes attacks of arthritis in people with high levels of uric acid in their blood. The hereditary form of gout is much more common in men. Gout caused by thiazide diuretics occurs equally in men and women. The first attack usually lasts a few days; a second attack may occur several months later. Treatment is with nonsteroidal anti-inflammatory drugs and other drugs (see page 130).

Crystals in the joints
The photograph below (magnified 28 times) shows the needlelike uric acid crystals that are found in the joints of people with arthritis caused by gout. Analysis of the joint fluid for crystals helps your doctor make a diagnosis.

Bacteria inside a joint
If your doctor suspects that you have an infection in a joint, he or she may remove a sample of synovial fluid through a needle inserted into the joint (see page 55). A smear of the synovial fluid on a glass slide, viewed under a microscope, will reveal the presence of any infective organisms, such as the staphylococcal bacteria shown here (magnified 1,400 times).

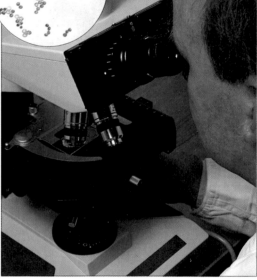

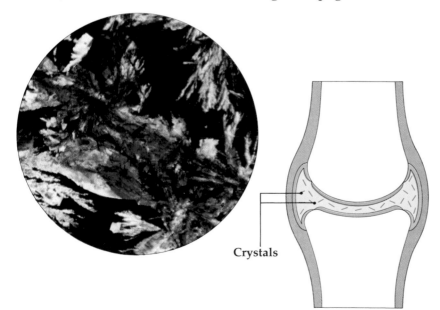

Crystals

ARTHRITIS CAUSED BY INFECTION

Arthritis may be caused by an infection, either directly or indirectly; in such cases, it is broadly referred to as infectious arthritis. In septic arthritis, bacteria or fungi from an infection elsewhere in the body enter the bloodstream and move into the joint, causing inflammation. In conditions such as reactive arthritis and Reiter's syndrome, an infection in some part of the body causes a generalized inflammatory reaction, which affects joints and other tissues.

Septic arthritis

Septic arthritis is usually caused by a bacterial infection of a joint; in rare cases, a fungus may be the cause. The condition tends to occur in people whose resistance to disease has been lowered by some other disorder and in people who already have joint damage (for example, from rheumatoid arthritis). Children are susceptible to septic arthritis when they have an infection caused by *Staphylococcus* or *Hemophilus* bacteria.

Bacteria from an infection in the body (such as a boil in the skin) may be carried in the bloodstream to a joint. Bacteria may also enter the joint directly after an injury. Typically, the person has shaking chills and a fever. The affected joint is swollen, warm, and painful, especially when it is moved.

Septic arthritis is diagnosed by analyzing samples of blood and synovial fluid. The condition is treated with antibiotics and by draining the infected synovial fluid from the affected joint.

Reactive arthritis

In cases of reactive arthritis, several joints become painful, inflamed, and swollen. These symptoms occur not as a result of direct infection but as a complication of the response of the body's immune system to an infection (usually a viral infection) such as infectious mononucleosis, hepatitis B, measles, and mumps. In most cases, the arthritis clears up in a few days without treatment and there is no permanent damage to the joints.

Reiter's syndrome

Reiter's syndrome is a potentially severe, chronic, intermittent condition occurring as a reaction to certain bowel or urethral infections. It is characterized by arthritis, conjunctivitis (inflammation of the transparent front covering of the eye), and urethritis (inflammation of the urethra). The arthritis usually starts in the feet, ankles, or knees. Nonsteroidal anti-inflammatory drugs such as aspirin are the main form of treatment for the painful symptoms and the inflammation caused by Reiter's syndrome.

JUVENILE RHEUMATOID ARTHRITIS

Juvenile rheumatoid arthritis is a rare, persistent arthritis that affects about one child in 1,000. It may affect only a few joints or many joints. The initial symptoms are often a limp or a reduction in joint function. Gradually, juvenile rheumatoid arthritis affects many joints and other body systems (see below). Wasting

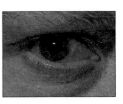

Conjunctivitis
Conjunctivitis (inflammation of the conjunctiva – the transparent front covering of the eye) is one of the recurring symptoms of Reiter's syndrome. Episodes of conjunctivitis are usually mild and clear up quickly.

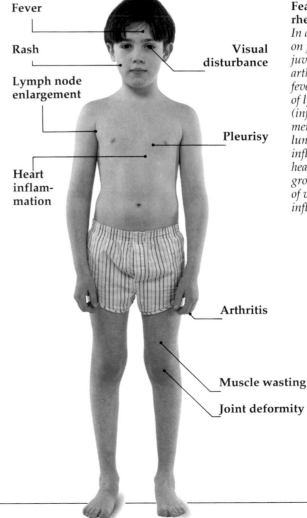

Fever

Rash

Lymph node enlargement

Heart inflammation

Visual disturbance

Pleurisy

Arthritis

Muscle wasting

Joint deformity

Features of juvenile rheumatoid arthritis
In addition to its effects on joints and muscles, juvenile rheumatoid arthritis may also cause fever, rash, enlargement of lymph nodes, pleurisy (inflammation of the membrane lining the lungs and chest cavity), inflammation of the heart, impairment of growth, and disturbance of vision caused by eye inflammation.

CASE HISTORY
A PAINFUL TOE JOINT

SINCE RETIRING FROM **playing professional golf, Carl had become a golf instructor at a nearby country club. One afternoon, after teaching a 3-hour class, he felt a slight twinge of pain in the big toe of his left foot. During the next 24 hours, the pain became so severe that he could not put any weight on his left foot. His wife drove him to the doctor's office.**

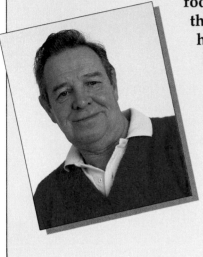

PERSONAL DETAILS
Name Carl Dell
Age 55
Occupation Golf instructor
Family Carl's father had gout and his grandfather had a severe form of arthritis affecting his foot, ankle, and knee.

MEDICAL BACKGROUND
Carl has always been in good health. He enjoys participating in a variety of sports. Carl had been to a cocktail party at the country club the night before the pain in his toe started.

THE CONSULTATION
While examining Carl's left foot, his doctor observes that the joint at the base of his big toe is inflamed, reddish purple, swollen, and warm. When the doctor gently moves the toe, Carl feels severe pain.

The doctor asks Carl some questions about his family's medical history. Carl tells his doctor that his mother never had any serious illnesses and died of heart failure at the age of 90; his grandfather had severe arthritis and his father had gout. Carl also remembers that his father had deposits of a white, crystalline substance on the upper edge of his ears.

The doctor takes a sample of Carl's blood and withdraws some fluid from the swollen joint of his big

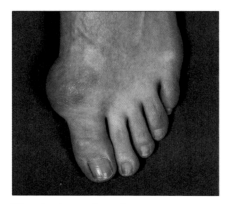

Classic signs of gout
During his acute attack, the joint at the base of Carl's big toe on his left foot became extremely painful and swollen, due to formation of uric acid crystals in the joint. White, crystalline deposits on the ears (right) due to uric acid crystal formation affect some people with gout.

toe. The samples are sent to a laboratory for examination. Carl's doctor prescribes indomethacin, a nonsteroidal anti-inflammatory drug.

THE DIAGNOSIS
Carl returns to his doctor 2 days later. He tells the doctor that his big toe feels much better. Carl's doctor tells him that the results of the tests have confirmed his suspicion that Carl has FAMILIAL GOUT, an inherited condition in which crystals of uric acid form in the joints and other tissues. The level of uric acid in his blood is higher than normal and the joint fluid sample, when examined under a microscope, contained needlelike crystals of uric acid. The crystals cause attacks of arthritis in joints, and repeated attacks may damage the joints. He warns Carl that drinking alcohol, being overly tired, and consuming foods such as sardines or organ meats sometimes trigger an acute attack.

THE TREATMENT
The doctor tells Carl to take the indomethacin for 7 to 10 days and to have the prescription refilled if another attack occurs.

THE OUTCOME
Carl's painful symptoms clear up with the indomethacin. He is able to return to teaching golf at the country club several days later.

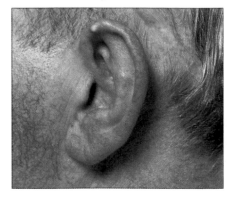

of the muscles and joint deformity may occur. Treatment of juvenile rheumatoid arthritis is similar to that of rheumatoid arthritis (see TREATING RHEUMATOID ARTHRITIS on page 86).

ARTHRITIS ASSOCIATED WITH OTHER DISEASES

Arthritis can be a major symptom of some diseases, such as systemic lupus erythematosus. For other diseases, such as inflammatory bowel disease and the skin disease psoriasis, arthritis occurs only in some cases.

Systemic lupus erythematosus

Systemic lupus erythematosus is a disorder of the body's immune system that affects other body systems. In addition to the general symptoms of fever, tiredness, and weight loss, most people also have arthritis that affects many of their joints, particularly joints in the hands. Other symptoms may include rash, anemia, mental disorder, pleurisy (inflammation of the lining of the lungs and chest wall), and kidney problems.

Treatment usually includes nonsteroidal anti-inflammatory drugs (such as aspirin) and corticosteroid drugs. Occasionally, other antirheumatic drugs, immunosuppressant drugs, or a combination of both may be prescribed.

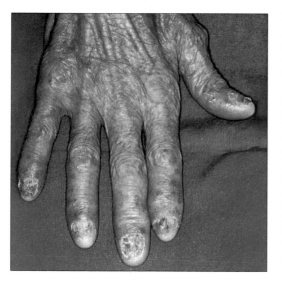

INFLAMMATORY BOWEL DISEASE

The cause of inflammatory bowel disease, which includes ulcerative colitis and Crohn's disease, is unknown. In ulcerative colitis, the inner lining of the colon becomes inflamed; in Crohn's disease the wall of the digestive tract is inflamed and becomes thickened. About 20 percent of people with these bowel disorders also have arthritis. The knees, ankles, and wrists are most commonly affected. Corticosteroid drugs are sometimes prescribed to treat both the inflammatory bowel disease and the arthritis.

Psoriatic arthritis
Arthritis develops in about 7 percent of people who have the skin disease psoriasis (thickened patches of red, inflamed skin). The joints of the fingers are most commonly affected; most people have pitting of the nails (shown at left). In some people, the arthritis develops before the psoriasis. Treatment of psoriatic arthritis is similar to that of rheumatoid arthritis (see TREATING RHEUMATOID ARTHRITIS *on page 86).*

ASK YOUR DOCTOR
JOINT DISORDERS

Q Our doctor says that my husband has pseudogout of his knee. Is this the same as gout?

A Not exactly. Pseudogout causes symptoms that are similar to those of gout, but the cause of pseudogout is slightly different. Gout is caused by deposits of uric acid crystals in a joint, usually in the big toe. Pseudogout is caused by deposits of calcium pyrophosphate crystals, usually in the knee. Pseudogout is most common in older people, especially after a major illness.

Q What causes Lyme disease? Does this disease cause permanent damage to the joints?

A Lyme disease is caused by a bacterium transmitted by the bite of a tick. A rash and flulike symptoms usually occur, followed (after weeks or months) by intermittent arthritis (periods of arthritis, followed by periods of remission). In most cases, the arthritis eventually goes away. Treatment with antibiotics, if given early enough in the course of the disease, can usually prevent the development of arthritis.

Q I have recently been told that I have rheumatoid arthritis. Is this the same as rheumatic fever?

A No, rheumatoid arthritis and rheumatic fever are different conditions. Rheumatoid arthritis is a form of inflammatory arthritis, the cause of which is unknown. Rheumatic fever starts after an infection with certain types of streptococcal bacteria and may affect the heart, skin, and brain, as well as the joints throughout the body. Rheumatic fever is no longer common in the US.

JOINT INJURIES

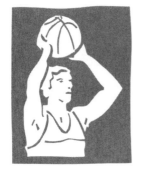

EACH JOINT IN YOUR BODY is designed to allow a certain range of motion. If a joint is moved beyond its normal range of motion or if a joint is forced to move in an unnatural direction, the structures in and around it (such as the joint capsule or ligaments) may be damaged. The severity of the damage depends on how the injury occurred and the strength of the force that caused the injury.

Injury is a common cause of damage to joints, and there are many different types of joint injury. People who exercise vigorously have a particularly high risk of damaging a joint, but even everyday activities such as walking can lead to injury, especially if you are overweight or if you are walking on uneven surfaces. Vigorous repetitive movements of a joint may cause painful inflammation of one of the joint tendons or of the outer covering of a tendon (see TENDON INJURIES on page 105).

Spraining your ankle
The joint most commonly sprained is the ankle. A sprained ankle is caused by rolling over onto the outside of your foot, putting your full body weight on the ligaments on the outside of your ankle. This may occur in a fall or when walking on uneven ground.

LIGAMENT INJURIES

An injury in which the joint is twisted or moved beyond its normal range of motion may cause stretching and sometimes tearing of one or more of the ligaments that support the joint. The injury is described as a strain if the ligament is simply overstretched, a sprain if the ligament is overstretched enough to tear some of its fibers, and a tear if the damage is so severe that the ligament is partially or completely severed. A torn ligament may lead to dislocation or subluxation (partial dislocation) of the bones in the joint that the torn ligament supports (see page 98). Symptoms of ligament injuries include pain that is made worse by moving the joint and tenderness, swelling, and instability of

Ligament sprain
A sprain is caused by overstretching and partially tearing the fibers of one or more ligaments that support a joint (below).

Symptoms of a sprain include bruising and painful swelling. Your doctor may take an X-ray of the injured joint to make sure that there is no fracture.

Fibula

Tibia

Sprained ligament

the joint. Black-and-blue discoloration of the skin over the joint (which is caused by bleeding under the skin) may appear after the injury.

Treatment of a strain or sprain includes four basic elements – rest, ice, compression, and elevation – known as RICE (see page 103). Your doctor may prescribe a nonsteroidal anti-inflammatory drug such as aspirin to reduce the pain and swelling. In some cases, your doctor may apply an elastic bandage to compress the injured area or apply a splint and tell you to keep the injured

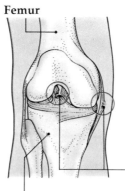

Femur

Ligament tear
A ligament tear is a severe injury in which one or several ligaments of a joint are partially or completely severed. Symptoms include painful swelling, limitation of movement, and stiffness.

Torn ligaments

Tibia

INJURIES THAT CAUSE JOINTS TO LOCK

Some joint injuries can cause the joint (particularly the knee joint) to "lock" in one position, which often causes severe pain. Loose bodies (sometimes called "joint mice") are detached fragments of cartilage or small pieces of bone inside the joint capsule. If the loose bodies become trapped between the bone ends, they can cause the joint to lock.

Gentle movement of a joint by your doctor will sometimes unlock the joint. However, if you have a severe injury or experience recurrent locking of a joint, arthroscopic surgery to repair the damage may be needed (see page 99).

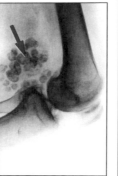

Loose bodies
If loose bodies in a joint (arrow) become lodged between the bone ends, they cause the joint to lock. The locking is usually temporary, but pain and swelling often last for several days.

Cartilage tears
A flap of free cartilage in your knee can become trapped between the bone ends (arthroscopic view shown at right). This causes your knee to lock, making it impossible to straighten your leg.

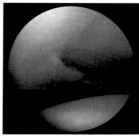

Tearing a knee ligament
A torn knee ligament is a common sports injury. The tear is caused by forceful overstretching of the ligament. This injury may occur if you twist your knee during an activity such as playing basketball or skiing.

limb elevated until the pain and swelling subside. Your doctor may suggest an exercise program designed to strengthen the joint and prevent future injuries.

Treatment of a severely torn ligament consists of either immobilizing the injured joint in a cast for at least 6 weeks or surgery to repair the torn ligament (see SURGICAL PROCEDURES on page 99).

SYNOVITIS

Synovitis is inflammation of the thin membrane (called the synovial membrane) that lines the inside of a joint capsule. The inflammation leads to an increased production of lubricating fluid from the synovial membrane, causing the joint to become swollen, painful, and often warm and red. Synovitis can be caused by injury, overuse, or infection

MONITOR YOUR SYMPTOMS
PAINFUL JOINTS IN CHILDREN

In children, pain in one or more joints is usually the result of a minor fall or injury. However, if the pain is severe or lasts a long time, it may indicate an underlying condition that needs medical attention. If you are at all uncertain about the cause of your child's pain, call your pediatrician immediately.

Joint pain may be generalized or localized in one area.
Is only one joint affected?

NO

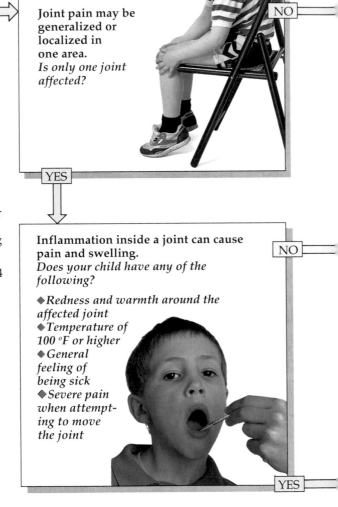

YES

BEGIN HERE

Injury is a common cause of joint pain in children.
Has your child recently fallen or been involved in sports activities?

NO

A soft-tissue injury (damage to the muscles, ligaments, or tendons around the joints) may be causing the pain.

Action For the first 24 hours, treat the affected area with ice packs and apply an elastic bandage or splint to the affected limb (or support an arm in a sling). Your child should rest the injured limb for several days. Elevate an injured foot, leg, or ankle whenever possible. Call your doctor if the pain persists with no improvement after 24 hours.

Inflammation inside a joint can cause pain and swelling.
Does your child have any of the following?

NO

◆ *Redness and warmth around the affected joint*
◆ *Temperature of 100 °F or higher*
◆ *General feeling of being sick*
◆ *Severe pain when attempting to move the joint*

YES

YES

NO

The severity of the pain may indicate the type of injury.
Is the affected joint or limb misshapen or is the child unable to move the joint or any part of the injured limb?

YES

EMERGENCY
CALL FOR MEDICAL HELP IMMEDIATELY!

A fracture or dislocation of the joint may be the cause of the pain.

Action Keep the child warm and as still as possible until medical help arrives. Do not try to manipulate the joint or move the child. Support the injured limb with a pillow, several sheets of folded newspaper, or other splinting material. Treatment will depend on the site and severity of the injury.

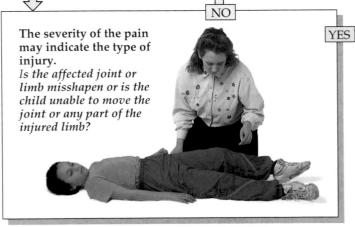

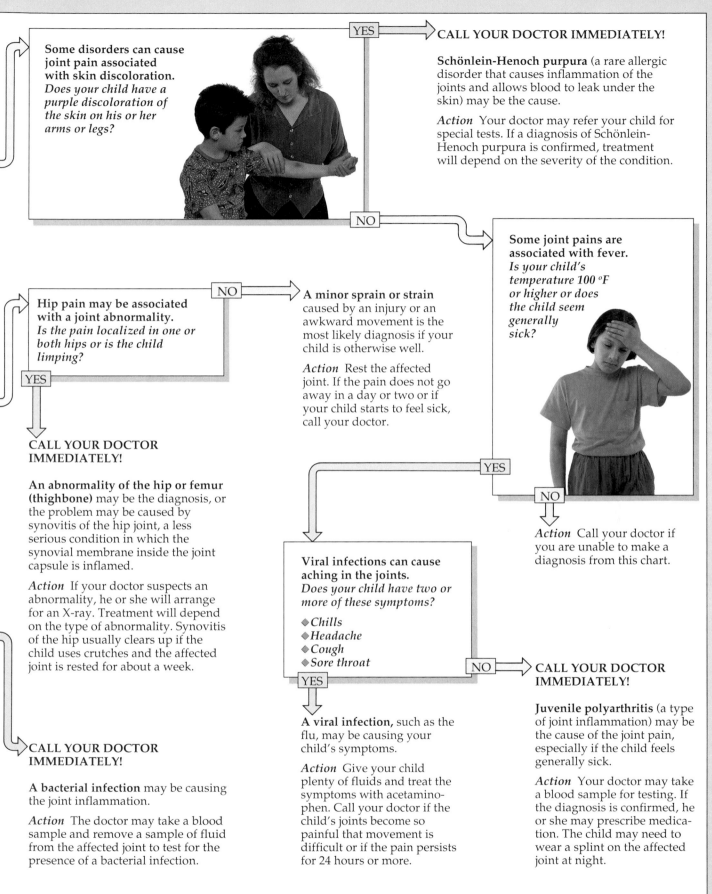

Some disorders can cause joint pain associated with skin discoloration. *Does your child have a purple discoloration of the skin on his or her arms or legs?*

YES → **CALL YOUR DOCTOR IMMEDIATELY!**

Schönlein-Henoch purpura (a rare allergic disorder that causes inflammation of the joints and allows blood to leak under the skin) may be the cause.

Action Your doctor may refer your child for special tests. If a diagnosis of Schönlein-Henoch purpura is confirmed, treatment will depend on the severity of the condition.

NO →

Some joint pains are associated with fever. *Is your child's temperature 100 °F or higher or does the child seem generally sick?*

Hip pain may be associated with a joint abnormality. *Is the pain localized in one or both hips or is the child limping?*

NO → A minor sprain or strain caused by an injury or an awkward movement is the most likely diagnosis if your child is otherwise well.

Action Rest the affected joint. If the pain does not go away in a day or two or if your child starts to feel sick, call your doctor.

YES →

YES

NO

Action Call your doctor if you are unable to make a diagnosis from this chart.

CALL YOUR DOCTOR IMMEDIATELY!

An abnormality of the hip or femur (thighbone) may be the diagnosis, or the problem may be caused by synovitis of the hip joint, a less serious condition in which the synovial membrane inside the joint capsule is inflamed.

Action If your doctor suspects an abnormality, he or she will arrange for an X-ray. Treatment will depend on the type of abnormality. Synovitis of the hip usually clears up if the child uses crutches and the affected joint is rested for about a week.

Viral infections can cause aching in the joints. *Does your child have two or more of these symptoms?*

◆ *Chills*
◆ *Headache*
◆ *Cough*
◆ *Sore throat*

YES

NO → **CALL YOUR DOCTOR IMMEDIATELY!**

Juvenile polyarthritis (a type of joint inflammation) may be the cause of the joint pain, especially if the child feels generally sick.

Action Your doctor may take a blood sample for testing. If the diagnosis is confirmed, he or she may prescribe medication. The child may need to wear a splint on the affected joint at night.

CALL YOUR DOCTOR IMMEDIATELY!

A bacterial infection may be causing the joint inflammation.

Action The doctor may take a blood sample and remove a sample of fluid from the affected joint to test for the presence of a bacterial infection.

A viral infection, such as the flu, may be causing your child's symptoms.

Action Give your child plenty of fluids and treat the symptoms with acetaminophen. Call your doctor if the child's joints become so painful that movement is difficult or if the pain persists for 24 hours or more.

of a joint; arthritis; or a disorder of the body's immune system.

Synovitis caused by an injury is treated by resting the joint. Your doctor may prescribe a nonsteroidal anti-inflammatory drug such as aspirin. Excess fluid inside the joint may be aspirated (removed from the joint through a needle) and a corticosteroid drug injected to reduce the inflammation.

Hemarthrosis

A hemarthrosis is a collection of blood inside a joint. It may occur after an injury or be caused by a defect in the blood's ability to form clots. The joint becomes swollen, stiff, and painful. Applying an ice pack helps reduce the swelling. Your doctor may apply a splint to immobilize the joint. You should elevate and rest the joint for several days.

DISLOCATION

A dislocation is a joint injury in which two normally opposing bone surfaces are displaced. In addition to severe pain and restriction of movement, dislocation causes swelling that makes the joint look misshapen. Call your doctor or a local emergency room immediately. Never try to reposition a dislocated joint yourself, because you could damage nerves or blood vessels or make an accompanying fracture worse. After your doctor repositions the bones, he or she will immobilize the joint until the surrounding soft tissues heal (usually in 3 to 6 weeks). When the soft tissues have healed, your doctor may recommend strengthening exercises.

Dislocating your elbow
A common site for dislocation is the elbow joint. Dislocation can result from a direct blow to the elbow or from falling onto an outstretched hand, which may occur when falling off a bicycle. A dislocation causes severe pain and tenderness.

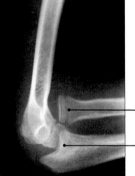

NORMAL

— **Humerus**

— **Radius**

— **Ulna**

— **Dislocated bones**

Repositioning the bones
Your doctor will reposition the bones after administering a general or local anesthetic. He or she may also aspirate blood (remove the blood through a needle) from the site of the dislocation. After the dislocated bones have been repositioned, the joint is immobilized with a cast or a splint to allow the damaged tissues around the joint to heal.

The injury
Bones of the elbow joint (above left) are displaced from their normal position (above right). A dislocated elbow requires immediate repositioning because it can damage nerves and blood vessels. Any damage can cause numbness in the arm and hand and bleeding. Dislocations can recur because joint tissues are permanently stretched and weakened. Surgery may be needed to stabilize the joint by tightening surrounding ligaments.

SURGICAL PROCEDURES
ARTHROSCOPIC REPAIR OF A SHOULDER INJURY

Arthroscopy **is a procedure used to diagnose and treat a variety of joint disorders. The inside of the damaged joint is examined through an arthroscope, a viewing tube with a tiny television camera at its end. If treatment is required, surgery can often be performed using instruments that are inserted into the joint through other incisions. The surgeon monitors the operation on the television screen.**

In the operating room
Arthroscopy allows the surgeon to examine the inside of the injured joint and avoids the large incisions usually used in conventional surgery. It also eliminates the time a patient must stay in the hospital, since arthroscopic surgery is performed in the outpatient surgical suite. During surgery for a shoulder injury, a general anesthetic can be given or a local nerve block can be administered to numb only the shoulder tissues.

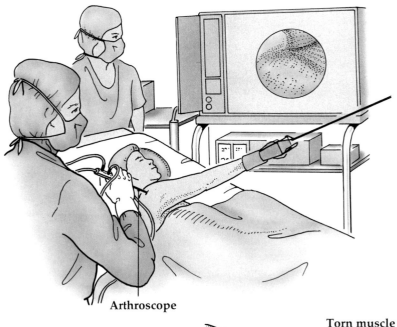

Arthroscope

1 The patient's arm is elevated by traction to give the surgeon access to the injured shoulder joint. The surgeon determines the most appropriate site to make a small incision for insertion of the arthroscope. One of three sites is usually chosen – on the back, the front, or the side of the shoulder, depending on the location of the injury. When a local anesthetic is used, epinephrine is injected along with the anesthetic to reduce bleeding and to facilitate insertion of the arthroscope through the small incision in the skin.

Traction

Shoulder joint

2 When the arthroscope is in position inside the joint, the other end is connected to a television monitor. The surgeon examines the joint structures for damage on the television screen. Surgery can be performed to repair the damage by inserting instruments into the shoulder through other incisions.

Torn muscle

Arthroscope

3 When the arthroscope is removed, the incisions are closed with sutures, metal clips, or adhesive tape, and a sterile dressing is applied. For about 3 days, a sling is used to support the shoulder; after that, gentle strengthening exercises can be started. Recovery time depends on the severity of the injury and the extent of the surgery that was performed to repair damage.

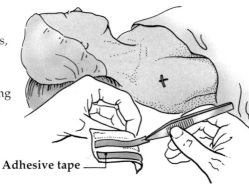

Adhesive tape

BURSITIS

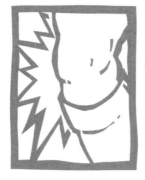

BURSITIS IS AN INFLAMMATION of a fluid-filled sac (called a bursa) around a joint. The inflammation causes pain and tenderness (and sometimes swelling) that is often aggravated by movement of the affected joint. Bursitis tends to develop in people who repeatedly place a lot of pressure on one particular joint, such as carpet layers or roofers who must kneel for long periods of time.

Symptoms of bursitis
When a bursa becomes inflamed, it fills up with excess fluid and produces pain or swelling, or both (below). The skin overlying the bursa may feel warm and look redder than normal.

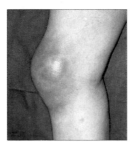

Throughout your body, there are dozens of fluid-filled sacs, known as bursae. Each bursa is like a cushion, either taking the pressure off the surface of a bone or reducing the friction around a tendon or muscle when it is stretched across a moving joint. In bursitis, a bursa becomes inflamed and swollen with excess fluid. This condition usually occurs as the result of damage to or irritation of the bursa caused by inflammation or infection of adjacent tissues, prolonged pressure on a joint, an injury to a joint, or forceful repetitive movement of a joint.

TYPES OF BURSITIS

"Housemaids' knee" is a bursitis that develops at the front of the kneecap, caused by prolonged kneeling in a crouched position on a hard surface. "Clergymen's knee" is inflammation of the bursa that lies below the kneecap and over the top of the shinbone, caused by kneeling in a more upright position.

Olecranon bursitis of the elbow is caused by prolonged pressure on the elbow against a desk or table.

Bursitis of the knee
Bursitis of the knee may develop in people who spend much of their working day kneeling. People who kneel for extended periods should wear knee pads to reduce the pressure on the bursae located at the front of and below the kneecaps.

Olecranon bursitis
The olecranon is the bony projection at the tip of the elbow. Olecranon bursitis of the elbow (also called students' elbow) causes pain, tenderness, and noticeable swelling at the tip of the elbow.

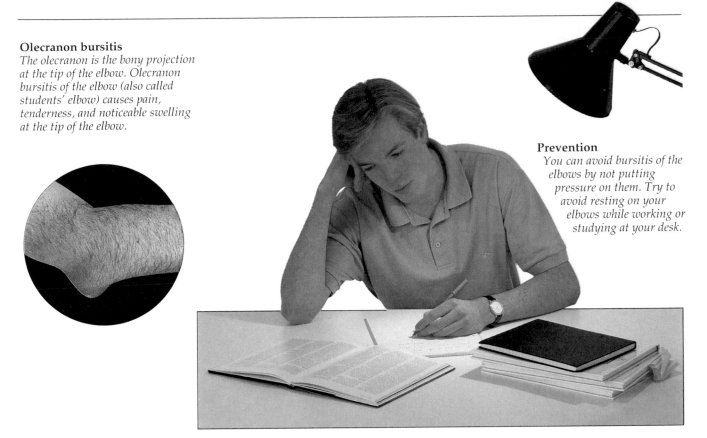

Prevention
You can avoid bursitis of the elbows by not putting pressure on them. Try to avoid resting on your elbows while working or studying at your desk.

Bursitis can occur as a complication of a deformity of the joint at the base of the big toe. A thickened, inflamed bursa, called a bunion, forms over the joint (see ASK YOUR DOCTOR on page 65). Pressure on the bursa around the heel bone from tight shoes can also cause bursitis.

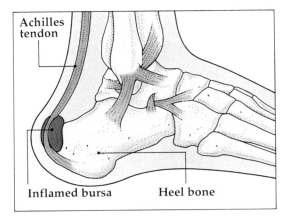

Bursitis in the heel
Bursitis in the heel is caused by direct pressure on the bursa around the heel bone. It is especially common in people who run long distances in shoes that do not fit properly. Also common in runners is Achilles bursitis, which develops at the point where the Achilles tendon attaches to the heel bone.

Treatment of bursitis

Bursitis often subsides if the affected part of the body is rested for a few days. Rest allows the excess fluid inside the bursa to be reabsorbed into the bloodstream. Use of an ice pack and taking a nonsteroidal anti-inflammatory drug such as aspirin can help ease discomfort and reduce inflammation.

If the inflammation persists, the fluid inside the bursa may need to be aspirated (removed through a needle). Your doctor will then apply a pressure bandage to prevent the fluid from re-forming. If the bursa looks infected or if the fluid removed shows signs of pus, your doctor will prescribe antibiotics. If there is no evidence of infection, a corticosteroid drug may be injected into the bursa to reduce the inflammation.

Although these treatments are usually effective, swelling and inflammation sometimes return. If this condition occurs repeatedly, a minor operation (called a bursectomy) may be performed to remove the affected bursa.

BURSECTOMY

Surgery to remove a bursa (called a bursectomy) is usually an outpatient procedure unless the swelling is very large, or the bursa is infected and the infection appears to be spreading. An incision is made over the top of the bursa and the bursa is removed. The incision is closed and a pressure dressing is applied. If the swelling is large, a drain may be placed in the incision for a few days to prevent buildup of fluid. After a bursectomy, the joint is usually put in a splint and should be rested in an elevated position for several days.

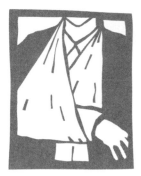

MUSCLE AND TENDON INJURIES

MUSCLES ARE ATTACHED to bones by tendons. The muscles and tendons in your body work together as units to produce movements of your skeleton. Muscle and tendon injuries are usually caused by athletics but may also occur in the course of your everyday activities. Damage can occur in the muscle or tendon itself, in the area where a muscle connects to a tendon, or in the area where a tendon attaches to bone.

Muscle or tendon injury may be caused by a sudden movement (such as twisting or stretching), a direct blow, or repetition of a movement over a prolonged period.

CRUSH INJURIES

An injury that crushes a muscle or muscles may temporarily weaken or even paralyze the damaged muscles. If damage to the muscles is not severe, normal muscle power returns slowly without treatment. However, crushed muscle fibers release a pigment, called myoglobin, into the bloodstream. If many muscles of the body are crushed, the large amounts of myoglobin and other substances released may damage the kidneys and cause kidney failure.

MUSCLE INJURIES

Excessive stretching of a muscle during any form of physical activity can damage its fibers, resulting in a muscle strain (overstretching of the muscle or tearing of some of the muscle fibers – also called a pulled muscle) or tear (overstretching that tears a large number of the muscle fibers; see below). These injuries cause pain, tenderness, swelling, and often painful spasms of the damaged muscle. Determination of the most appropriate treatment depends on the type and severity of the injury.

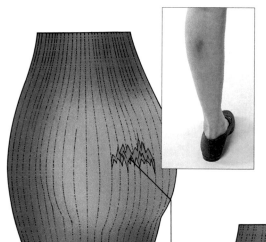

Torn muscle fibers

Muscle strain
If only some of the muscle fibers are torn, the injury is called a muscle strain. Bleeding inside the damaged muscle causes pain, tenderness, swelling, and often painful muscle spasms. A bruise frequently appears in the skin over the muscle a few days after the injury.

Torn muscle fibers

Bleeding

Muscle tear
When a large number of muscle fibers are torn, the injury causes bleeding, severe pain and tenderness, and swelling. If a tear is very severe, an indentation in the muscle may be visible. When there is considerable bleeding, an accumulation of blood can form a clot (called a hematoma). Your doctor may aspirate the hematoma (remove the blood clot through a needle) from the muscle tear.

RICE: FIRST-AID TREATMENT OF MUSCLE AND JOINT INJURIES

If you have a muscle or joint injury, it is easy to perform the correct first-aid treatment for the first 48 hours after the injury by remembering the acronym RICE (rest, ice, compression, elevation). If you are concerned about your condition, call your doctor. Proper first-aid treatment will help reduce the pain and swelling caused by the injury and will also help you recover more quickly.

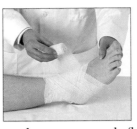

Compression
Wear a compression bandage around the injured muscle or joint for at least 2 days to reduce bleeding and swelling. If you use an elastic bandage on an injured muscle or joint, apply pressure evenly (but not tightly), starting below the injury and working upward. Apply the bandage over a thin pad of cotton to allow for additional swelling. Make sure that you extend the bandage well above and below the injury. If the bandage causes numbness, tingling, or pain, or if the skin below it turns white or blue, it is too tight and should be loosened immediately.

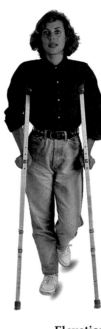

Rest
Rest the injured muscle or joint and avoid placing any unnecessary weight on it or moving it. Rest reduces the amount of bleeding from damaged blood vessels inside an injured muscle, minimizes the risk of further damage to the muscle or joint, and allows time for the tissues to heal. You can rest an injured muscle of the shoulder, elbow, arm, or hand in a sling. If you have injured a leg muscle or sprained your ankle, use crutches to keep your weight off the leg when you stand or walk.

Elevation
Keep an injured limb raised above the level of the heart as much as possible. Elevation facilitates the drainage of fluid from the damaged muscle and helps reduce the amount of bleeding and swelling. Elevate your arm or hand with a sling. If you have an injured muscle in your leg, keep your foot elevated, either by lying flat with the foot and calf supported by pillows or cushions, or by sitting with the foot resting on a stool.

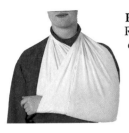

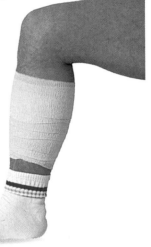

Ice, not heat
Apply an ice pack to the injured muscle or joint for up to 10 minutes at a time (or until the area becomes numb or red) every few hours, for the first 48 hours. Ice relieves pain by numbing nerve endings inside the injured tissues. Ice also limits swelling and bruising by reducing the amount of bleeding from damaged blood vessels. Never soak an injured muscle or joint in hot water or use a heating pad within the first 48 hours.

The first-aid treatment of a muscle injury is described on page 103. In addition to the standard treatment of rest, ice, compression, and elevation (known as RICE), your doctor may recommend taking a nonsteroidal anti-inflammatory drug such as aspirin. When a muscle strain or tear heals, scar tissue forms inside the muscle. Gentle stretching exercises begun about 48 hours after your injury will help minimize the amount of muscle shortening caused by the scar tissue. Once these stretching exercises no longer cause any pain, you can begin muscle strengthening exercises. A severe muscle tear may require surgery.

A blood clot in a muscle

A strong physical force against a muscle may cause severe bleeding and formation of a hematoma (a blood clot) inside the muscle. This causes swelling, pain and tenderness, muscle spasms, and bruising. A common site of a muscle hematoma is the quadriceps muscle of the thigh, sometimes resulting from being kicked in the front of the thigh.

First-aid treatment of a muscle hematoma is the same as that used for muscle strains and tears. If a muscle hematoma has developed, it is very important to rest the muscle for the first 48 hours and not begin exercising too soon.

MUSCLE CRAMPS

A cramp is a brief, painful contraction of a muscle. The cause of muscle cramps is largely unknown. However, fever, hot weather, or excessive or prolonged contraction of a muscle during exercise can cause muscle cramping; the excessive loss of sodium salts through perspiration interferes with normal functioning of muscles.

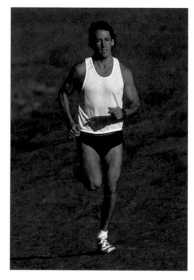

How exercise causes cramping
During moderate exercise, muscles receive an adequate supply of oxygen from the blood. One cause of muscle cramping is thought to be related to an inadequate supply of oxygen to the muscle during prolonged exercise. The sustained muscle contraction that occurs during prolonged exercise tends to restrict the flow of blood (which carries oxygen) through the muscle. Another factor contributing to cramping is thought to be the buildup of chemical waste products produced by the exercising muscles.

Night cramps
Cramping in the leg muscles at night may be the result of poor circulation of blood; chemicals produced in the muscles during daytime physical activity are not efficiently dispersed during the night and cause cramping. Treatment of night cramps includes massaging and stretching the cramping muscles. Your doctor may recommend calcium or quinine, which may relieve or prevent night cramps.

CAUSES OF MUSCLE SPASMS

In addition to the type of muscle cramps that often occur with exercise, several types of injury and disorders of the brain and nervous system can cause painful spasms (prolonged, painful contraction of a muscle).

Bleeding in a muscle

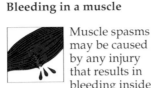

Muscle spasms may be caused by any injury that results in bleeding inside the muscle tissues from damaged blood vessels. The bleeding stimulates an involuntary contraction of the muscle fibers. A muscle strain or tear can cause bleeding in a muscle.

Damage to other structures

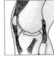

Muscle spasms may be caused by injury of structures underneath the muscle, such as dislocation of a joint or displacement of a disc of cartilage in the spine. The damage to other structures may irritate the nerve that supplies a muscle and trigger the painful spasms.

Brain and nervous system disorders

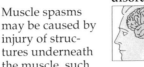

Muscle spasms may be caused by brain and nervous system disorders, such as stroke, multiple sclerosis, and cerebral palsy. In these disorders, the muscle spasms are caused by abnormal nerve signals that are sent to muscles, sometimes from the spinal cord instead of from the brain.

MUSCLE STIFFNESS

Strenuous physical activity may cause your muscles to feel stiff and sore for several days. These symptoms are caused by minor damage to some of the muscle fibers and by residual waste products produced in the muscle that have not been absorbed into your bloodstream.

You can reduce muscle stiffness by performing warm-up and cool-down exercises before and after your workout (see page 31). If you still feel stiff and sore for some time after an exercise session, avoid vigorous exercise until your muscles have recovered to prevent a more serious injury to your muscles.

TENDON INJURIES

Tendon injuries include tears in the tendon fibers, inflammation of a tendon (tendinitis), and inflammation of the covering of a tendon (tenosynovitis).

Tendon tears

A tear of a tendon is usually the result of a sudden, strong contraction of the muscles that stretch the tendon; the tear may be partial or total. A torn tendon causes pain, tenderness, and swelling. There may be deformity caused by a displaced muscle near or at the site of injury.

Minimizing muscle stiffness
Before vigorous exercise, warm up with a gentle stretching and loosening-up routine. This will reduce the severity of any muscle stiffness and soreness. Follow vigorous exercise with a cool-down routine, using some of the same exercises you used to warm up. A cool-down routine keeps the blood flowing through the muscles and helps disperse waste products produced by your muscles during exercise.

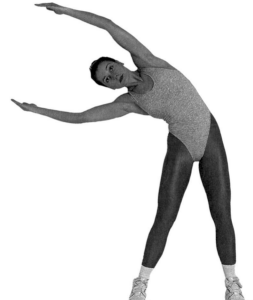

Baseball finger
If you try to catch a baseball with your fingers pointed toward the ball, the force of the ball hitting your fingertips can tear the tendons that straighten your fingertips. Your doctor may immobilize your fingers with a splint or insert a wire through the bones to keep your fingers straight while the tendons heal. Healing of the torn tendons may take several months.

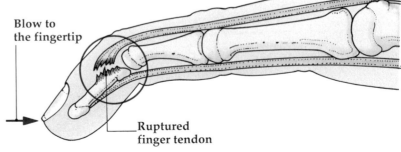

Blow to the fingertip

Ruptured finger tendon

SURGICAL PROCEDURES
REPAIRING A TORN ACHILLES TENDON

A TORN ACHILLES TENDON **is often treated by an operation to reattach the torn ends of the tendon. Surgery is usually performed while the patient is under general anesthesia and takes about an hour to complete. An overnight hospital stay is usually required and complete recovery takes at least 3 months.**

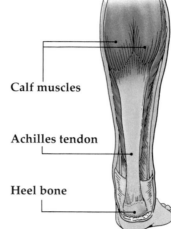

Achilles tendon
The Achilles tendon connects the calf muscles to the heel bone. When the calf muscles contract, they raise the heel off the ground by pulling on the Achilles tendon. A torn Achilles tendon, in addition to causing pain, tenderness, and swelling, usually results in a visible gap in the tendon and makes it impossible to raise the heel of the injured leg off the ground.

Calf muscles

Achilles tendon

Heel bone

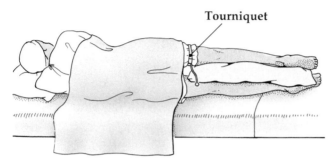

Tourniquet

1 The patient is given a general anesthetic. For the surgeon to repair the torn Achilles tendon without blood obscuring the injury, a tourniquet is placed around the thigh of the injured leg. This procedure blocks the entry of blood to the lower part of the leg.

2 A member of the surgical team cleans the foot and calf with an antiseptic. The surgeon makes an incision about 3½ inches long down the back of the calf and exposes the torn ends of the Achilles tendon.

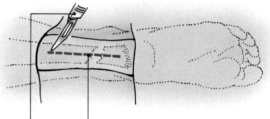

Scalpel   Incision

3 The surgeon removes any blood clot and damaged tissue lying between the torn ends of the tendon. He or she bends the patient's knee and points the toes downward to relax the calf muscles and to bring the ends of the tendon together. The surgeon then stitches the ends of the torn tendon together. In some cases, an additional piece of tissue, such as the tendon from another muscle in the calf (the plantar muscle), is stitched around the reattached ends of the torn tendon to reinforce the repair.

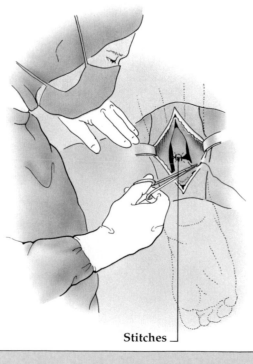

Stitches

4 The surgeon then stitches the incision closed and applies a dressing. The lower part of the leg is immobilized in a cast that extends above the knee. The knee is slightly bent, the foot points downward, and the toes are exposed.

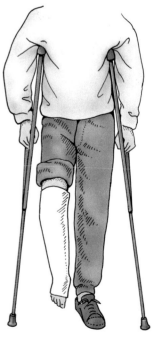

A tendon usually attaches a muscle to a bone so when a tendon is torn the muscle becomes detached from the bone.

A strong contraction of the calf muscles, which can occur during a sprint or if you suddenly go up onto your toes to reach an overhead tennis shot, may tear the Achilles tendon (see page 106).

The long tendon of the biceps muscle in the upper part of the arm can tear when you lift a very heavy object. In most cases, physical therapy to strengthen the other muscles in the upper part of the arm prevents significant loss of function caused by this injury.

Tendinitis

Inflammation of a tendon – called tendinitis – is usually caused by excessive friction between the outer surface of the tendon and a bone. Tendinitis causes pain, tenderness, and, sometimes, restricted movement of the muscle that is attached to the tendon.

Tendinitis may be treated with nonsteroidal anti-inflammatory drugs (such as aspirin), ultrasound treatment (use of high-frequency sound waves to reduce inflammation and speed healing), and corticosteroid injections. If movement remains restricted, an operation may be performed to remove fibrous bands that have formed around the tendon.

Tenosynovitis

Some tendons of the hands, wrists, feet, and ankles are enclosed in a fibrous tissue – the tendon sheath – that allows the tendon to slide over a joint. In tenosynovitis, the inner lining of a tendon sheath becomes inflamed. Symptoms include pain, tenderness, and swelling. You may hear a grating noise or feel a crackling sensation when the tendon is moved.

Tenosynovitis is usually treated with a nonsteroidal anti-inflammatory drug (such as aspirin) or corticosteroid injections. Repeated injections of a corticosteroid drug (more than four in 1 year) may weaken the tendon and predispose it to tearing. The affected hand or foot may be immobilized for a few weeks. If movement of the affected hand or foot becomes restricted, surgery may be required.

Injuries causing tenosynovitis
Tenosynovitis usually affects the tendons in the hand and wrist. It may occur in people whose jobs involve repetitive hand movements.

Tendons

Tendon sheaths

Tendinitis in the shoulder
Inflammation of the supraspinous tendon in the shoulder is caused by friction that occurs between that tendon and a bony edge (the acromion process) on the shoulder blade each time the arm is raised above the head. This injury is common in people who play a lot of racket sports.

Acromion process of shoulder blade

Inflamed supraspinous tendon

Muscle

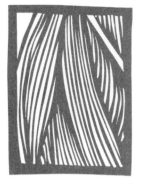

MUSCLE DISORDERS

I**F YOUR MUSCLES ARE NOT USED** regularly, such as when you are confined to bed, the muscles tend to atrophy (shrink or waste away). A muscle may also shrink if its nerve supply is cut off; this can happen when an injury severs a nerve. A number of rare musculoskeletal diseases also cause wasting and weakness of the muscles. Muscle weakness and wasting often develop in people with widespread cancer or severe heart failure.

Muscle weakness and wasting are the most common symptoms of a muscle disorder. Pain, stiffness, spasms, tenderness, and swelling of the muscles are other symptoms of muscle disease.

SHRINKING OF UNUSED MUSCLES

Muscles that are not used for a prolonged period of time will atrophy (shrink or waste away). People with fractures who must stay in bed for more than a few days may notice weakness and wasting of their muscles. Exercise helps prevent and reverse muscle wasting.

Prolonged weakness and nonuse of muscles may result in contractures (permanent shortening of muscles and tendons) and stiffness of the joints. To prevent contractures, your doctor may recommend an exercise program, application of heat, and massage. If a contracture develops, surgery may be needed.

STRENGTHENING YOUR LEGS

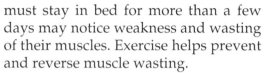

If you have been confined to bed for more than a few days, you may find that your legs feel weak. The following exercise will help strengthen the quadriceps muscle in the front of your thigh. The exercise should be done once or twice each day. After a few days you should notice an improvement in the strength of your thigh muscles.

1 Lie on your back on your bed or on the floor.

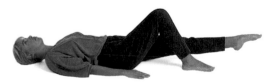

2 Lift your left leg a few inches off the bed or floor, keeping the opposite knee flexed. Hold your leg up while you count slowly to 10. Repeat the leg lift four or five times. Then do the exercise using your right leg.

HORMONE AND MINERAL DISORDERS

To function normally, muscles need minerals, nutrients, and hormones delivered by the bloodstream. If the amounts of hormones or minerals are abnormally high or low, the muscles may be damaged. Myopathy (degeneration of muscle) is often first apparent as weakness in the thighs and the upper parts of the arms. Difficulty climbing stairs or rising from your chair without pushing yourself up with your arms may be a symptom of muscle weakness.

Muscle weakness may be caused by abnormal levels of calcium or potassium in the blood, diabetes mellitus, a disorder of the thyroid gland, or an excess of corticosteroid hormone resulting either from an adrenal gland disorder or from taking a corticosteroid drug for a long period of time for a condition such as asthma. Muscle weakness may also develop as a result of abnormal production of hormones by some lung cancers.

Warning sign of a hormone or mineral disorder
The first sign of a hormone or mineral disorder is often difficulty climbing stairs, caused by weakness of the muscles in the thighs.

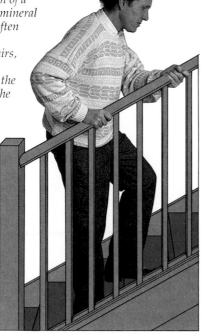

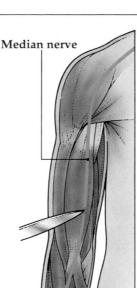

Median nerve

A stiff arm
If nerve cells in areas of the brain that control motor functions are damaged (as the result of a stroke, for example), muscles that are controlled by those areas of the brain become weak and stiff. However, muscle wasting is only slight. Physical therapy is useful in helping to restore muscle strength and function after a stroke.

Nerve cell damage in the brain

A nerve supplying arm muscles

Forearm muscles

A floppy arm
If a nerve is damaged, the muscles supplied by that nerve become weak, floppy, and noticeably wasted. For example, a knife injury that severs the median nerve in the upper part of the arm affects muscles in the forearm and around the thumb and some of the fingers.

Thumb and finger muscles

However, muscle weakness is rarely the first, or only, sign of any of these conditions; each condition usually causes various other symptoms before becoming severe enough to affect the muscles.

The strength of a muscle that has become weakened as the result of any illness usually returns spontaneously when the underlying condition is treated or has healed. Exercising the affected muscle may speed up strengthening.

MUSCULAR DYSTROPHY

The muscular dystrophies are a group of relatively rare, often inherited diseases that cause weakness and atrophy (shrinking or wasting away) of muscles.

Your doctor may suspect the diagnosis of muscular dystrophy from your

---

DRUGS AND MUSCLE WEAKNESS

Some drugs, such as prednisone, cause loss of potassium and protein and may cause muscle weakness, usually after prolonged treatment. The muscle weakness sometimes lessens after use of the drug is stopped. Exercising the affected muscles usually helps speed up strengthening. Abuse of alcohol can also cause muscle weakness.

CASE HISTORY
AN INHERITED MUSCLE DISORDER

Rosalyn was pleased when her friends began to compliment her on how slender her figure had become. But she was also concerned because she had noticed that she seemed to be walking more slowly than before and, when taking an exercise class, she had difficulty getting up off the floor. She decided to see her doctor.

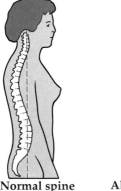

PERSONAL DETAILS
Name Rosalyn Blair
Age 27
Occupation Bookkeeper
Family Grandfather and one aunt had a disabling muscle disorder. Both of these relatives died in their late 50s.

MEDICAL BACKGROUND
Rosalyn had the usual childhood illnesses and suffers from hay fever. She has never had any serious medical problems and has seen her doctor only three or four times during the past few years for her hay fever.

Making the diagnosis
The doctor notices that, when Rosalyn stands, the lower part of her back has an exaggerated inward curve (lordosis). A muscle biopsy sample (right) shows degeneration of muscle fibers, confirming the diagnosis of muscular dystrophy.

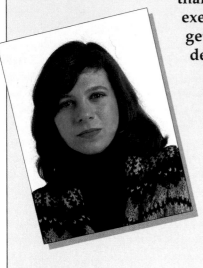

Normal spine   Abnormal lordosis

THE CONSULTATION
Rosalyn tells her doctor that she now has trouble getting up from sitting on the floor and she can't seem to walk as fast as she used to. Her doctor asks her about her family's medical history, and she tells him that her

Healthy muscle fibers

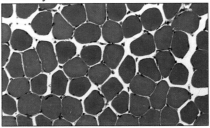

Degenerated muscle fibers

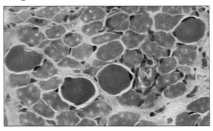

grandfather and an aunt had serious muscle disorders. He examines her, looking for muscle atrophy (shrinking or wasting away of muscle) and checking her reflexes, posture, and the strength of her muscles. The muscles around her pelvis and hips show signs of atrophy and are weak. The reflexes of her elbows and knees are weak. Rosalyn's spine shows an exaggerated inward curvature (called lordosis) in the lower part of her back. Her doctor also notices that she walks with a waddle.

FURTHER INVESTIGATION
Rosalyn's doctor tells her that he is fairly sure she has a form of inherited muscle disorder but explains that he would like to perform a few more tests to determine the type of disorder. He takes a sample of blood to check for the enzyme creatine kinase, which is released from affected muscles. He also performs electromyography (a test to determine the electrical activity of muscle and the conduction of nerve impulses) and a muscle biopsy (removal of a small sample of muscle tissue for examination under a microscope).

THE DIAGNOSIS
Rosalyn's tests indicate that she has LIMB-GIRDLE MUSCULAR DYSTROPHY, an inherited disorder of the muscles in the shoulders and pelvis.

THE TREATMENT
Rosalyn's doctor explains that there is no cure for limb-girdle muscular dystrophy, which causes progressive deterioration of muscles. He tells her that stretching exercises to prevent contractures (permanent shortening of muscles and tendons of a joint), exercises to maintain muscle function, and occasionally wearing a brace can help her lead as normal a life as is possible with this muscle disorder.

symptoms, signs of muscle atrophy, family history, and various tests.

There is no treatment for the underlying muscular weakness of muscular dystrophy, but some people benefit from stretching exercises or surgical release of contractures (permanent shortening of the muscles and tendons of a joint) to maintain the ability to walk. Equipment is available to increase comfort and function for people with muscular dystrophy.

Weakness in Duchenne type muscular dystrophy
Because their legs are weak, children with muscular dystrophy get up from the floor by "climbing up" their legs, pushing with their hands against their ankles, knees, and then their thighs.

Duchenne type muscular dystrophy

Duchenne type muscular dystrophy is the most common form of the disease and occurs almost exclusively in boys. Although born with the genetic defect that causes the disease, affected boys do not usually have symptoms before age 3. The initial signs of muscle weakness may be falling frequently or difficulty getting up from the floor, climbing stairs, or keeping up with friends.

By age 5, the muscles usually have become noticeably weak and may appear enlarged, particularly the muscles of the hips and legs. By age 12, many chil-

dren with the disease cannot walk. During the early teenage years, the disease progresses further and may involve the respiratory muscles and the heart. Scoliosis (spinal curvature) may occur because of spinal muscle weakness. In the past, few people with Duchenne type muscular dystrophy survived their teen years, usually dying of an acute lung infection. Today there are good prospects for effective treatment.

MYASTHENIA GRAVIS

Myasthenia gravis is a rare disorder caused by a lack of response, or a diminished response, of muscles to nerve impulses. When nerve impulses stimulate a muscle, they cause the release of a chemical called acetylcholine. The acetylcholine must attach to a receptor on the muscle cell to stimulate contraction of the muscle. In people with myasthenia gravis, the body's immune system produces antibodies that attack the acetylcholine receptors. The transmission of nerve impulses to a muscle is impaired, and muscles become weak.

Effects of myasthenia gravis
In myasthenia gravis, the muscles of the face and eyes often become weak; drooping eyelids and double vision may be the first signs of the disease. Weakness of the muscles of the throat may cause difficulty speaking and swallowing. The illustration below right shows the principal muscles affected. Later, the muscles in the arms and legs may also be affected. The degree of muscle weakness varies from day to day and worsens rapidly with exercise. About 10 percent of people with myasthenia gravis that begins later in life have tumors of the thymus gland (shown below).

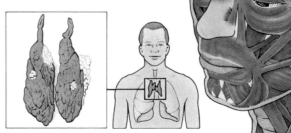

Thymus gland

MYOTONIC DYSTROPHY
The characteristic feature of this inherited disorder is an inability to relax muscles after contraction. A person with myotonic dystrophy has difficulty relaxing his or her hand after grasping an object. Symptoms develop between ages 20 and 30. The muscles of the face, neck, hands, and feet may become weak. Cataracts may develop at an early age, and the heart may be affected. There is no specific treatment, although some medications can be used to ease the inability of muscles to relax. Most people eventually become severely disabled.

Principal muscles affected in the early stages

CASE HISTORY
LOSS OF MUSCLE STRENGTH

KATHY HAD THOUGHT FOR SOME TIME that her arm and hip muscles seemed to be getting weaker. She had been having increasing difficulty getting up out of her chair in the library, where she had been spending a lot of time on her work. She also began to find it difficult to type for more than a few minutes. She made an appointment to see her doctor.

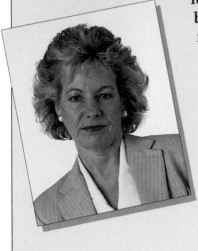

PERSONAL DETAILS
Name Kathy Bergstrom
Age 45
Occupation Literary historian
Family Both Kathy's parents are healthy.

MEDICAL BACKGROUND
Apart from fairly frequent colds and a mild case of the flu during the past winter, Kathy's medical history has been unremarkable.

THE CONSULTATION
Kathy's doctor examines her and tests her muscle strength. He finds she has weakness in the muscles of her shoulders, the upper part of her arms, her hips, and the upper part of her legs. He takes a blood sample to determine the cause of this muscle weakness.

FURTHER INVESTIGATIONS
The tests show that Kathy's blood is positive for rheumatoid factor and antinuclear antibodies, results that strongly suggest she has an autoimmune disorder (a disorder in which the body's immune system attacks its own tissues). The level of the enzyme creatine kinase in her blood is raised, indicating that muscle breakdown is occurring. Her doctor tells her that more tests are needed to make a diagnosis. Electromyography (a test to determine the electrical activity of a muscle and the conduction of nerve impulses) shows changes that indicate inflammation of the muscles. A muscle biopsy shows dead muscle fibers and many inflammatory cells.

THE DIAGNOSIS
The doctor explains that Kathy has POLYMYOSITIS – an inflammatory disorder that is affecting her muscles. The cause of the disorder is not known. The inflammatory cells infiltrating her muscles are lymphocytes (cells produced by the body's immune system) that are attacking and destroying the muscle fibers.

THE TREATMENT
Kathy's doctor prescribes the corticosteroid drug prednisone to be taken orally, initially in a dose of 50 milligrams each day. Within a few weeks she feels stronger. The dosage of prednisone is slowly decreased. The doctor tells Kathy that he will continue to monitor her condition and the effect of her medication.

THE OUTCOME
Kathy suffers no relapses and continues to get stronger over several months. The doctor tells her that he cannot predict how long the remission of her disease will last. If a relapse occurs, it will be treated by adjusting the dosage of her medication. Kathy's work is unaffected and she continues to spend long periods at her word processor working on her latest book.

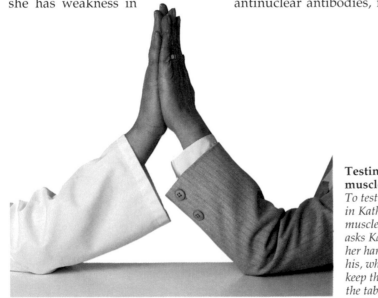

Testing muscle strength
To test the strength in Kathy's arm muscles, the doctor asks Kathy to push her hand against his, while they both keep their elbows on the table.

Myasthenia gravis is diagnosed by physical examination, review of the person's medical history, and various tests that measure the muscles' response to certain drugs. Treatment with drugs can be helpful (see page 138). The condition of some people with myasthenia gravis is improved by removing the thymus gland, which forms part of the body's immune system and is thought to be partly responsible for abnormal antibody activity. Temporarily removing antibodies from the blood by a process known as plasmapheresis is used in cases of sudden, severe deterioration or when a person who has myasthenia gravis is prepared for surgery.

POLYMYALGIA RHEUMATICA

Polymyalgia rheumatica is characterized by pain and stiffness in the muscles in the shoulders, neck, hips, and thighs. The disease usually develops in people over the age of 50; women are affected three times more commonly than men.

People with polymyalgia rheumatica feel generally sick. The onset of pain and stiffness in the muscles is usually rapid and may follow a flulike illness. Symptoms are usually most noticeable when awakening and after periods of inactivity. People with polymyalgia rheumatica typically describe late afternoon as their best time of day. They may also have temporal arteritis (inflammation of the arteries in the head and neck). Headaches caused by temporal arteritis may be severe. Arteries of the eye may become blocked, which results in sudden blindness.

TREATMENT OF TEMPORAL ARTERITIS

If your doctor suspects that you have temporal arteritis, he or she will order blood tests and a biopsy (removal of a small piece of tissue from the artery for examination under a microscope) to help confirm the diagnosis. Your doctor may prescribe a corticosteroid drug in a high dosage at first; then it will be reduced to a lower dosage. This treatment must be given as soon as possible because it is the only way that the risk of blindness can be avoided.

Effects of polymyalgia rheumatica
People with polymyalgia rheumatica often experience severe, painful morning muscle stiffness (mainly of the large muscles of the shoulders) and may find it difficult to get out of bed without assistance.

ASK YOUR DOCTOR
MUSCLE DISORDERS

Q I recently went to see my doctor because the upper part of my back aches. After he examined me thoroughly, he told me that I have fibrositis and prescribed medication. What is fibrositis?

A Fibrositis is a term for aches and pains, particularly in the muscles of the back and around the shoulder blades, sometimes with areas of tenderness. It may be accompanied by symptoms of depression. Other terms that are sometimes used are fibromyalgia and fibromyositis. Your doctor made his diagnosis by ruling out other more serious conditions. Fibrositis does not indicate any serious underlying disease and will not lead to significant disability. Treatment of fibrositis may include painkillers, antidepressants, application of heat, and massage.

Q My sister's son has Duchenne type muscular dystrophy. If she were to have another child, would he or she also be affected by the condition?

A Your sister is a "carrier" of Duchenne type muscular dystrophy. A carrier of this disease is a woman who has the gene for Duchenne type muscular dystrophy, and the risk of passing the disease on to her male children is 50 percent. The disease is not passed on to female children, but the female children of a carrier have a 50 percent chance of being carriers. The muscular dystrophy gene has been identified, and doctors can now determine whether a woman with a family history of muscular dystrophy is a carrier of the gene. New techniques in genetic testing have also made it possible to diagnose the condition before birth.

CHAPTER FIVE

BACK PAIN AND SPINAL DISORDERS

INTRODUCTION

BACK PAIN

SPINAL INJURIES AND DEFORMITIES

Back pain is the single most common symptom related to the bones, muscles, and joints and is often the reason why people go to see their doctors. It is one of the most common causes of working days lost due to illness. In some cases of back pain, a specific diagnosis can be made; in others there is no obvious cause for the back pain. Backaches for which the cause is uncertain (sometimes called "nonspecific" back pain) affect many people – at least one in every 50 adults. Nonspecific back pain may be caused by incorrect posture, which puts excess strain on your spine and causes muscles to go into spasm. Back pain may be triggered by an awkward or strenuous movement. The pain may develop slowly or occur suddenly, may be continuous, or may occur only when your back is moved into certain positions. Bending and twisting your

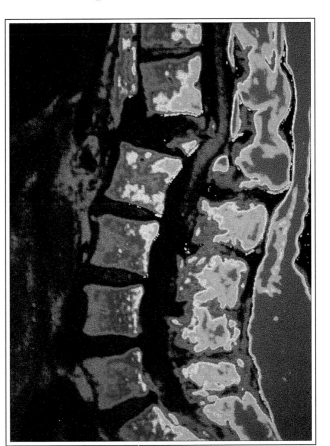

back or coughing and sneezing may aggravate the pain. Nonspecific back pain usually occurs in the lower part of the back, sometimes in one spot. Although a nonspecific backache may be very painful, it does not usually indicate a serious underlying problem. The pain usually lasts only a few days and may be relieved by rest and taking mild painkillers such as aspirin. However, nonspecific back pain does tend to recur.

You are more likely to have back pain if your job involves a lot of heavy lifting or carrying, if you spend long periods of time sitting in one position or bending awkwardly, or if you sleep on a sagging mattress. You are more prone to back pain if you are overweight or out of shape or if members of your family have a history of backache. Back pain also frequently occurs during a severe illness or the late months of pregnancy.

The most common causes of disorders affecting the cervical (neck) region of the spine are arthritis in the joints and degeneration of an intervertebral disc (a pad of cartilage located between two adjacent vertebrae), which may lead to prolapse (rupture) of the disc. The 33 vertebrae of the spinal column form a strong, protective casing for the spinal cord and contain channels through which nerves pass to and from the rest of your body. Injury or deformity of the spine may put pressure on the spinal cord or nerves, leading to muscle weakness and abnormal sensations such as numbness or tingling. Minor variations in the bony structure of the spine are common, especially in the lower part of the back, and may not cause any symptoms. Major abnormalities, injuries, and diseases of the spine cause pain and deformity and may damage the spinal cord and nerves.

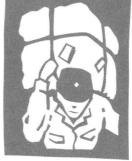

BACK PAIN

Y OUR SPINE IS A FLEXIBLE STRUCTURE that consists of 33 vertebrae, powerful muscles, shock-absorbing discs of cartilage between the vertebrae, and strong ligaments that bind the vertebrae together. Although your spine can withstand considerable stress and strain, an overload on one or more of the supporting structures of the spine or damage to the vertebrae can cause back pain.

Back pain varies from an aching discomfort that may be present for a short time after waking up and then again at the end of the day to a sudden, severe pain that makes it difficult or impossible to move. Back pain frequently occurs in the lower part of the back (called the lumbar region) because of the load placed on this area when we stand and walk.

ACUTE AND CHRONIC BACK PAIN

Back pain that occurs suddenly (called acute back pain) is usually caused by an injured ligament or muscle, resulting in muscle spasms. A less common cause of back pain is a prolapsed (ruptured) disc.

CAUSES OF BACK PAIN

Injured ligaments or muscles
An injury to the ligaments or muscles attached to the vertebrae may cause pain in one area of your back. Sudden, forceful movement or strenuous lifting may injure the ligaments and muscles in your back.

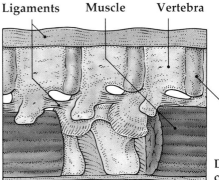

Ligaments   Muscle   Vertebra

Disc of cartilage

Muscle spasm
Damage to any of the structures of the spine – vertebrae, discs of cartilage, ligaments, or muscles – may cause a muscle to go into spasm, resulting in pain. Muscle spasms may cause your back to pull over to one side and cause movement to be painful and restricted.

Viral infections and stomach, heart, and lung disorders
Back pain is a common symptom of a viral infection such as the flu. Disorders of the stomach, heart, and lungs can also cause pain in the upper part of the back. An enlarging aortic aneurysm (a balloonlike swelling of the walls of the aorta, the main artery from the heart) may also cause back pain between the shoulder blades.

Osteoarthritis
Persistent pain in your back may be caused by chronic disc degeneration, in which the discs of cartilage between the vertebrae become worn as a result of osteoarthritis (see page 78). Many people who have back pain have signs of osteoarthritis on an X-ray of the spine.

Acute back pain is often the result of lifting a heavy object or bending awkwardly. In many cases, acute back pain goes away in a few days. A more severe injury that damages one or more vertebrae is another cause of acute back pain. Severe spinal injuries are described in the next section (see page 122).

Chronic (persistent or recurring) back pain can often be attributed to being overweight or to an injury. However, it may also be caused by arthritis of the spine or a bone disease affecting the spine. Back pain may be a symptom of a disorder that is affecting the lungs, heart, major blood vessels, or kidneys.

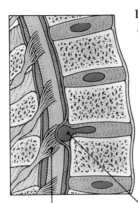

Spinal nerve root   **Prolapsed disc**

Disc prolapse (rupture)

Between each vertebra is a pad of cartilage called an intervertebral disc. Each disc has a hard, outer region and a soft center. Through wear and tear or pressure, the center may rupture and protrude through the outer layer of the disc (sometimes called a "slipped disc") and press on a ligament or on a spinal nerve root, causing back pain. The back pain becomes more severe when you cough or sneeze or strain on the toilet.

Sciatica

Sciatica is pain that radiates along the sciatic nerve. The pain extends from the buttocks down the back of the thigh and leg to the calf or foot. Sciatica is usually caused by a disc swelling or prolapse (rupture), putting pressure on the sciatic nerve or its roots.

Sciatic nerve

Sciatic nerve

Vertebra

Kidney infection

Pyelonephritis – infection of a kidney, usually the result of a urinary tract infection – may cause back pain. Symptoms of pyelonephritis include pain and tenderness in the side of the lower part of your back, fever, chills, and pain when urinating.

Intervertebral disc

Bone diseases and tumors

Bone diseases such as osteoporosis or osteomalacia are common causes of back pain. A less common cause of back pain is a tumor in the vertebrae or spinal cord.

Spinal abscess

A rare cause of back pain is an abscess (a collection of pus formed as the result of an infection) in the spinal canal – called an epidural abscess. An infection may affect the vertebrae and spread to the spinal canal, causing an abscess. The abscess may compress nerves, causing radiating pain, or may compress the spinal cord, causing loss of sensation and weakness or paralysis of the lower half of the body and loss of bladder and bowel control.

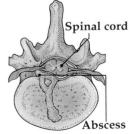

Spinal cord

Abscess

Ankylosing spondylitis

If you have back pain that becomes more severe after resting, with stiffness in your back and hips that lasts for hours, you may have ankylosing spondylitis (see page 119).

SELF-HELP FOR BACK PAIN

To relieve back pain, try resting in bed on a firm mattress or lying flat on the floor. Placing a pillow under the knees is not recommended for all people with back pain, especially for elderly people who are susceptible to deep-vein thrombosis (a blood clot in the veins located deep in the leg muscles). To relax your spine by elevating your legs, put pillows under your heels and calves. Avoid any position or movement that aggravates your back pain. When sitting, sit up straight and well back on the seat of a firm chair. When you get up from lying down or sitting, push up with your arms to reduce the stress on your spine.

Painkillers such as aspirin (or other nonsteroidal anti-inflammatory drugs) or acetaminophen usually help relieve pain. Heat treatment using a hot water bottle or a heating pad can help

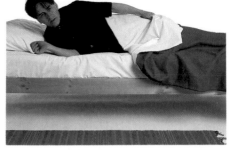
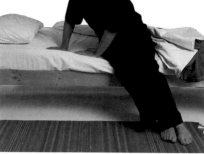

Getting out of bed
The most comfortable way to get out of bed is to roll onto your side toward the edge of the bed; then lower your legs to the floor while you raise the upper part of your body to a sitting position.

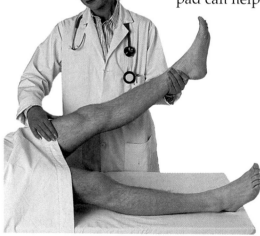

The physical examination
While you are standing, your doctor observes your posture and checks the range of motion in your back. While you are lying down, your doctor examines you for areas of tenderness and signs of muscle spasm. He or she raises your legs one at a time, keeping the knees straight, to see if movement is restricted by pain. The doctor also evaluates nerve and muscle function in both of your legs by looking for signs of weakness, checking for abnormal reflexes, and testing for loss of skin sensation.

relieve the muscle spasms or cramps that occur with chronic back pain. If heat doesn't seem to help, try an ice pack on the painful area for a few minutes.

It may take a few days for your back pain to go away. Even if your back pain is the result of a prolapsed (ruptured) disc, you can often recover completely without surgery.

TREATMENT BY YOUR DOCTOR

When you go to see your doctor about pain in your back, he or she will ask you about it and any other symptoms you may have. Your doctor will examine you and may arrange for you to have blood tests or X-rays. Treatment will depend on the cause of your back pain. Doctors usually recommend rest and sometimes mild painkillers (such as aspirin or other nonsteroidal anti-inflammatory drugs). Muscle relaxants are sometimes prescribed. Your doctor may also suggest back stretching and strengthening exercises. A lightweight brace to support your back, heat treatments and massage, or traction may be recommended. If severe pain persists, your doctor may inject a corticosteroid drug and an anesthetic into the lower part of your spine.

WHEN TO SEE YOUR DOCTOR

See your doctor if:

◆ Your back pain persists or recurs often.

◆ Your back pain is accompanied by weakness, numbness, or a tingling sensation in your legs.

◆ Your back pain is accompanied by loss of bladder or bowel control.

◆ You have severe back pain after a fall, in which case you should not try to move unless you are in immediate danger. You should be moved only by people who have training in administering first aid (see page 123).

CASE HISTORY
A PAINFUL, STIFF BACK

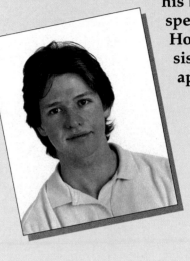

ANTHONY IS A LAW STUDENT and a member of his college's racquetball team. One morning after playing a very strenuous game of racquetball, Anthony awoke with pain and stiffness in the lower part of his back and in his buttocks. Assuming he had strained his back, he took some aspirin and spent the day studying in bed. However, when the pain persisted the next day, he made an appointment to see his doctor.

PERSONAL DETAILS
Name Anthony Fairbanks
Age 21
Occupation Law student
Family Anthony's father is healthy; his mother has had rheumatism in her back for many years.

MEDICAL BACKGROUND
Anthony has participated in sports since he was in grade school. He fractured his wrist at age 15.

THE CONSULTATION
Anthony's doctor examines his spine and finds that he cannot move his back much without pain. The examination reveals no numbness or tingling sensations or abnormal reflexes in his legs. His doctor concludes that Anthony may have strained his back and prescribes aspirin and bed rest. A week later, the stiffness and pain have not gone away. Anthony's doctor refers him to a rheumatologist, a doctor who specializes in arthritis and other conditions affecting the joints and connective tissues.

THE RHEUMATOLOGIST'S CONSULTATION
Anthony tells the rheumatologist that he has recently been feeling some stiffness in his back, but that it usually goes away after he exercises.

The rheumatologist examines Anthony and discovers that his spine has lost much of its flexibility. There is no tenderness around the vertebrae but pressing on Anthony's sacroiliac joints causes a considerable amount of pain. The doctor asks Anthony to take a deep breath and then exhale, and notes that the expansion of his chest is restricted.

Blood test results show evidence of an inflammatory condition, but are negative for rheumatoid factor, an antibody that is often present in people with rheumatoid arthritis. X-rays of Anthony's sacroiliac joints show that his joints are inflamed.

THE DIAGNOSIS
The rheumatologist tells Anthony that his low back pain and stiffness and the inflammation of the sacroiliac joints indicate that he has ANKYLOSING SPONDYLITIS, a condition in which the vertebrae and sacroiliac joints fuse. This disease usually starts before age 30 and is often mistaken in its early stages for a strained back.

THE TREATMENT
The rheumatologist prescribes aspirin and refers Anthony to a physical therapist. The therapist gives Anthony advice on how to maintain good posture and teaches him a variety of exercises and activities to help minimize his symptoms and prevent any disability in the future.

THE OUTLOOK
Because Anthony's condition has been diagnosed at an early stage, there is a good chance he will be able to lead a relatively normal life.

Normal bones

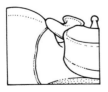

Fused bones

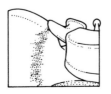

Sacroiliac inflammation
Inflamed sacroiliac joints (right) are characteristic of ankylosing spondylitis. After the initial inflammation of the joint, outgrowths of bone (called spurs) gradually develop on each side of the joint and fuse (left) so that the joint cannot be moved, a process known as ankylosis.

Ilium

Sacrum

Inflamed sacroiliac joints

SURGICAL PROCEDURES
MICRODISCECTOMY

MICRODISCECTOMY IS **an operation used to treat a prolapsed (ruptured) disc in the spine that is causing pain by pressing on a spinal nerve or nerve root. An incision is made in the skin and in the tissues over the disc. Using an operating microscope and special instruments, the surgeon removes the protruding parts of the disc. The operation leaves a relatively small scar and requires a few days' stay in the hospital.**

1 The patient is given an anesthetic and is positioned face down on the operating table. The surgeon inserts a needle into the spine at the level of the prolapsed disc, and an X-ray is taken to confirm the level. The surgeon marks the level of the disc and the site of the incision on the patient's skin.

2 The surgeon makes the incision. After deepening the incision through the underlying tissue, he or she inserts a retractor into the space between the vertebrae adjacent to the prolapsed disc.

3 Looking through the operating microscope, the surgeon inserts a cutting instrument called a rongeur and removes a portion of the ligament that connects the vertebrae. This action reveals the outer covering (the dura) of the nerves in the lower part of the spine and the compressed nerve root.

4 The surgeon uses a retractor to pull the nerve root aside to show the protruding disc underneath. He or she makes a small, cross-shaped incision in the fibrous covering of the disc.

5 The surgeon removes the protruding disc tissue in pieces with a rongeur and clears the center of the disc of any other loose material. The surgeon also removes any loose pieces of disc tissue that he or she can see or feel in the spinal canal.

6 After making sure that the nerve is no longer compressed, the surgeon removes the retractors and closes the incision. The patient can get out of bed the next day.

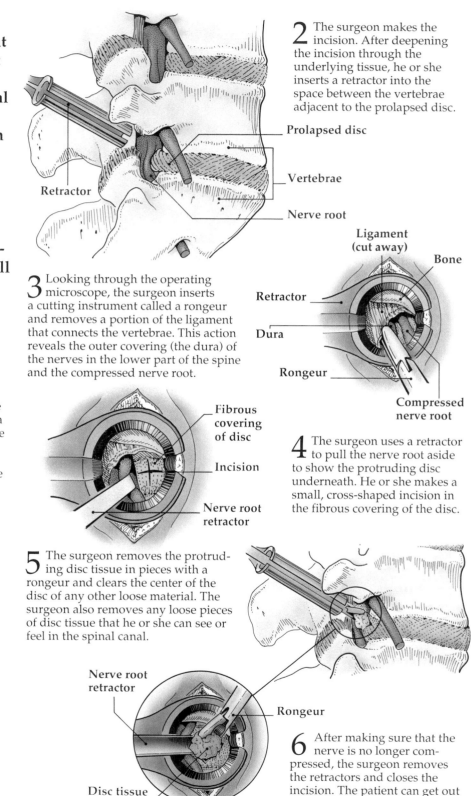

Retractor

Prolapsed disc

Vertebrae

Nerve root

Ligament (cut away)

Bone

Retractor

Dura

Rongeur

Compressed nerve root

Fibrous covering of disc

Incision

Nerve root retractor

Nerve root retractor

Rongeur

Disc tissue

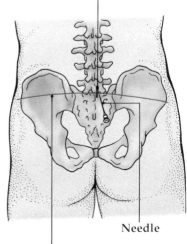

Site of incision

Needle

Level of disc prolapse

Traction

If your back problem is related to compression of a disc and the pain has not been relieved with mild painkillers and complete bed rest, your doctor may recommend spinal traction. Traction stretches your spine while you lie flat on your back; weights on a pulley system are attached to a harness fitted to your pelvis. Some doctors believe that traction is helpful. Others believe traction produces little or no improvement.

Treatment of disc prolapse

If back pain and sciatica are caused by a disc prolapse (rupture), bed rest is usually the best treatment. Applying heat to the painful area may also help relieve pain. If the pain persists for more than a few days, you should call your doctor. Your doctor may inject a corticosteroid drug into the area of the compressed nerve root or an anesthetic into the lower part of the spine to help relieve the pain.

If these treatments over a period of several weeks fail to relieve your pain, surgery is an alternative. Your doctor may remove a small piece of bone from a vertebra in order to relieve pressure on the compressed nerve root (a procedure called laminectomy) or, if several discs must be treated, spinal fusion may be performed (see page 127).

An alternate method of treating a mild, uncomplicated disc prolapse is chemonucleolysis. In this treatment, using X-ray guidance, your doctor injects an enzyme called chymopapain into the disc. Chymopapain dissolves the disc's soft center, causing the disc to shrink, thus relieving the pressure on adjacent nerve roots. Some people have a severe allergic reaction to chymopapain.

Treating bone cancer

Cancer in the bones of the spine is usually treated by radiation therapy or chemotherapy (anticancer drugs); a tumor involving the spinal cord is removed surgically, if possible.

NECK PAIN

If you wake up with a painful, stiff neck, it is usually the result of spasms of the muscles in your neck. The pain and stiffness usually go away in a few hours or days without treatment other than aspirin. A strain or a twisting injury of the neck causes painful spasms and tenderness of the neck muscles. A neck strain may occur gradually (for example, neck pain caused by holding your head in an awkward position for a long period of time) as well as suddenly. Neck pain and stiffness accompanied by a headache and fever may be due to a generalized viral infection. If you have neck pain caused by an injury or pain that has lasted for more than a few days, call your doctor.

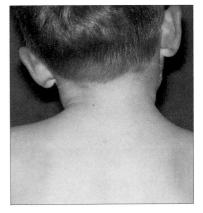

Torticollis
Torticollis is the result of severe spasms of muscles in the neck that twist the neck and tilt the head in an abnormal position. The neck is very painful and stiff. Muscle spasms may occur after a minor neck injury or may be the result of anxiety, sleeping in an awkward position, or an injury at birth. Treatment may include heat, ultrasound, or a soft foam collar. Torticollis caused by an injury at birth may require surgery.

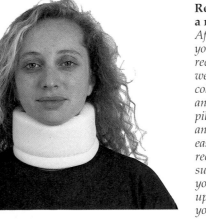

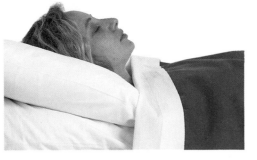

Recovery from a neck injury
After a neck injury, your doctor may recommend that you wear a soft foam collar during the day and sleep with two pillows until the pain and muscle spasms ease. During your recovery, try to avoid sudden movements of your neck, looking up or reaching above your head, carrying or lifting heavy objects, and sitting in one position for too long. Heat treatment and gentle massage often help relax muscle spasms.

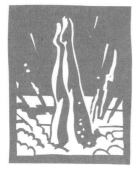

SPINAL INJURIES AND DEFORMITIES

AN INJURY TO THE SPINE may damage not only the bones and joints of the spinal column but also the spinal cord. Damage to the spinal cord and spinal nerves can cause paralysis (loss of movement) and loss of sensation below the level of the injury. Deformity of the spine may be caused by an injury, a birth defect, or a disease that affects the spinal vertebrae or muscles.

Stable injuries
In stable fractures and dislocations, the alignment of the vertebrae and attachments of the ligaments remain intact, preventing abnormal movement between the vertebrae. Damage to the spinal cord or spinal nerves is uncommon. Stable injuries may be caused by a compression force through the longitudinal axis of the spine or by a moderate force that flexes the spine.

The most common types of spinal injuries are a broken spine (caused by diving into shallow water or a motorcycle or automobile accident) or damage to the spinal cord (caused by gunshot wounds). It is important to know when to suspect that a spinal injury may have occurred and how to provide the proper first-aid treatment, if necessary, for this type of injury (see page 123).

SPINAL INJURIES

Many spinal injuries cause only slight pain and bruising, but serious injuries may fracture or dislocate the vertebrae. Whether a fracture or dislocation is stable or unstable (see illustrations below) is an important factor in your doctor's determination of treatment.

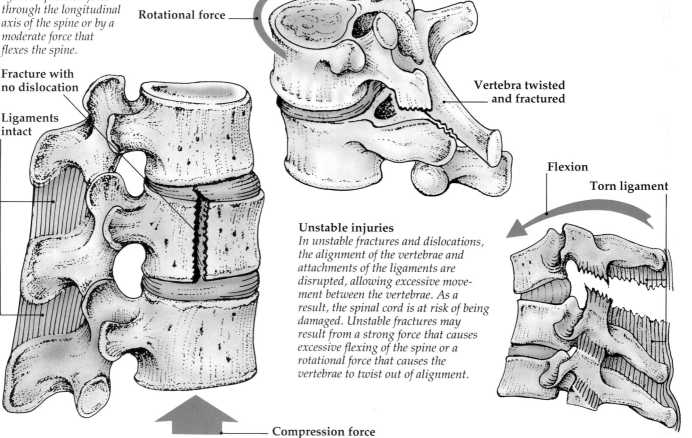

Rotational force

Vertebra twisted and fractured

Fracture with no dislocation

Ligaments intact

Flexion

Torn ligament

Unstable injuries
In unstable fractures and dislocations, the alignment of the vertebrae and attachments of the ligaments are disrupted, allowing excessive movement between the vertebrae. As a result, the spinal cord is at risk of being damaged. Unstable fractures may result from a strong force that causes excessive flexing of the spine or a rotational force that causes the vertebrae to twist out of alignment.

Compression force

Divisions of the spine
The spine has five sections – the cervical region (in the neck), the thoracic region (in the chest), the lumbar region (in the lower part of the back), the sacrum (between the hipbones), and the coccyx (the tailbone). Back injuries usually occur in the cervical, thoracic, and lumbar regions of the spine.

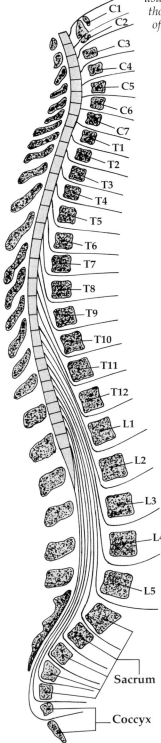

C1
C2
C3
C4
C5
C6
C7
T1
T2
T3
T4
T5
T6
T7
T8
T9
T10
T11
T12
L1
L2
L3
L4
L5
Sacrum
Coccyx

The cervical spine
There are seven cervical vertebrae, each connected by a series of joints that allow your head to bend forward, backward, and sideways and to rotate. The vertebrae or joints may be injured if their normal range of motion is exceeded or if stress is applied along the longitudinal axis of the spine, as would occur if you fell onto the top of your head.

The thoracic spine
The thoracic spine consists of 12 vertebrae. A pair of ribs attaches to each vertebra. The ribs help stabilize this region of the spine and make it resistant to injury. The most common injuries in this area are those that crush the vertebrae.

The lumbar spine
There are five vertebrae in the lumbar spine, located in the lower part of the back between the lowest pair of ribs and the top of the pelvis. This region of your spine is relatively mobile and bears the weight of your head, chest, and abdomen, which makes it susceptible to injury. The most common injury in the lumbar spine is a crush fracture of a vertebra.

Cervical spine injury
Damage to the spinal cord and nerves commonly occurs with injuries of the cervical (neck) region of the spine. Severe injury may cause total paralysis (total loss of movement) and total loss of sensation below the level of the injury. A less severe injury may result in partial paralysis and partial loss of sensation.

Severe injury at or above the fourth cervical vertebra may be immediately fatal. If the injury is not fatal, it often destroys the nerves that stimulate the muscles needed to breathe; mechanical ventilation (use of a machine to take over breathing) is needed.

Diagnosis and treatment
Your doctor will examine you to evaluate the severity of your injury, ensuring that your neck stays immobilized during the examination. X-rays, CT scanning (see page 50), or MRI (see page 48) provide detailed images of your injury.

If the fractured cervical vertebrae are out of alignment, traction may be used to realign the vertebrae. One method of traction uses tongs securely placed on each side of the skull; weights are attached to the tongs to pull gently on the neck. The person's body weight acts as a counterforce. A halo vest may also be used for fractures of the cervical vertebrae (see illustration at right).

Unstable injuries to the cervical spine may be treated by an operation to fuse the vertebrae at the level of the injury (see page 127). After the operation, the neck must be supported. A soft foam collar may provide sufficient support. In more severe injuries, a brace may be needed; the brace is usually worn for a few months.

Many people with severe nerve damage spend time at rehabilitation centers to help them adapt to their disability.

FIRST AID FOR A SPINAL INJURY
If you suspect someone may have a spinal injury, do not move the person without medical assistance unless the person is in a life-threatening situation. Moving the head, neck, or back can damage the spinal cord. If the person must be moved before medical help arrives, immobilize the neck and back. Place a wide board behind the head, neck, and back, keeping them aligned. Tie the board around the forehead, under the armpits, and across the lower abdomen. When moving the person, do not let his or her body bend or twist.

Halo-vest traction
Fractures of the cervical spine may be treated by halo-vest traction.

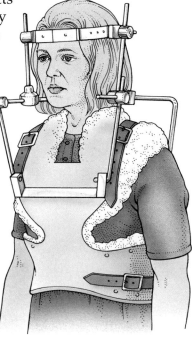

CASE HISTORY
BACK PAIN AFTER A FALL

WHILE VISITING HER DAUGHTER'S **family, Barbara tripped on her granddaughter's teddy bear and fell down the stairs. She was able to get up and seemed to be in no pain. However, Barbara quickly became aware of a severe pain in the middle of her back. Her daughter helped her get into bed and called the doctor.**

PERSONAL DETAILS
Name Barbara Brandeis
Age 58
Occupation Freelance fabric designer
Family Barbara's father died of a heart attack. Her mother recently fractured her hip.

MEDICAL BACKGROUND
Barbara is a petite woman who lives a very sedentary life. She has been treated for only minor ailments. Barbara went through the menopause at age 53 and has had no apparent postmenopausal problems.

THE CONSULTATION
The doctor notes that Barbara's fall has caused some bruising in the small of her back. Gently touching the bruised part reveals an area of severe tenderness. The doctor suspects Barbara's fall may have caused damage to her spine and arranges for Barbara to have X-rays taken of the lower part of her back.

THE DIAGNOSIS
Barbara's X-rays show that she has a significant reduction of bone density, a condition called osteoporosis that is caused by loss of bone protein and minerals. Osteoporosis often occurs in women after the menopause. The doctor tells her that she has a CRUSH FRACTURE of one of her vertebrae. The impact of her fall compressed a vertebra and caused it to collapse. She has also fractured small structures on two other vertebrae. Since these fractures appear to be stable, there should be no danger of any of the fractured bones moving out of position.

THE TREATMENT
The doctor prescribes a painkiller and a mild tranquilizer and tells Barbara to rest in bed on a firm mattress for 2 weeks. The doctor prescribes hormone replacement therapy for the osteoporosis, which may slow further loss of bone density. Barbara's daughter asks her mother to stay at her house while she recuperates; Barbara agrees.

THE OUTCOME
When the pain caused by the fractures has eased, Barbara starts doing the gentle exercises the doctor has instructed her to do while she rests in bed to help keep her muscles in good condition. These exercises also reduce the increased rate of mineral loss from bone that occurs during prolonged bed rest. After 2 weeks, Barbara's pain has almost disappeared and she returns to see the doctor. The doctor assures her that the fractures are healing and she will not have to wear the brace needed by some people who have had similar types of falls. She continues to exercise to improve the mobility of her spine, which feels a little stiff. As she gets stronger, she is able to increase the intensity of the exercises.

THE FOLLOW-UP
Barbara soon feels better. As soon as she is able, she starts to take walks several times a week. The only remaining trouble with her spine is occasional stiffness in the morning.

Barbara's exercises
This gentle side-bending exercise helps restore the mobility of Barbara's spine.

CERVICAL STRAIN OR SPRAIN

The ligaments, muscles, discs of cartilage, and joints of the cervical spine (the neck area) may be injured if the neck is forcefully bent backward or forward. Neck injuries usually involve a strain or minor sprain of neck ligaments. The main symptoms of an injury to the cervical spine are neck pain and stiffness, with aching across the shoulders and down the arms. Symptoms may not become apparent for 6 to 12 hours after the injury. Your doctor may recommend taking analgesic drugs (painkillers) and wearing a soft foam collar for a few days.

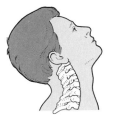

Hyperextension injury
If a vehicle is hit from behind, the occupant's head is suddenly thrown backward, and the neck is hyperextended (bent backward to a greater than normal degree).

Car headrests
The use of properly adjusted car headrests can prevent or greatly reduce the severity of hyperextension injuries.

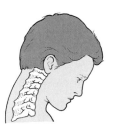

Flexing injury
If a vehicle is hit head-on, the occupant's head is thrown forward and the neck is flexed (bent forward). The chin hits the chest, which restricts the forward movement of the neck.

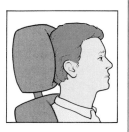

Crush and burst fractures

In a crush fracture, the front part of a vertebra collapses. This type of injury is often caused by a fall. A much less severe force may cause a crush fracture in a person with osteoporosis (loss of protein and minerals from bone).

Crushing of a vertebra causes localized back pain. Damage to the spinal cord and nerves rarely occurs. If a lumbar vertebra is severely crushed, the lumbar spine loses its normal curvature.

A burst fracture is a variant of a crush fracture. While a crush fracture is caused by pressure through the long axis of the

Crush fracture
A crush fracture is caused by pressure on the spine when it is flexed. The spinal vertebrae are made of spongy bone that compresses, rather than cracks, when subjected to pressure.

spine when it is flexed, a burst fracture is caused by pressure on the spine when it is straight. Burst fractures often cause damage to the nervous system.

Treatment

A moderately severe crush fracture is usually treated by bed rest and exercises to help maintain mobility. In some cases, a spinal brace may be needed in the first few weeks after the injury. Burst fractures may require a longer period of bed rest or surgery to ensure stability of the spine. Treatment of severe fractures and dislocations of the lumbar spine is similar to the treatment of cervical injuries.

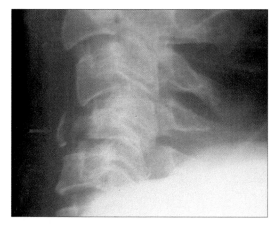

Burst fracture
In a burst fracture, the vertebra is pushed outward as shown in the X-ray above. Bony fragments or disc material may be forced out from between the vertebrae or into the spinal canal.

FIRST AID FOR A NECK INJURY

If you suspect someone may have a neck injury, do not move the person without medical assistance unless the person is in a life-threatening situation. Any movement of the head can result in paralysis or death. If the person must be moved before medical help arrives, immobilize the neck with a rolled towel, sweater, or newspaper about 4 inches wide wrapped around the neck and tied loosely in place. Position a wide board behind the head and back, extending down to the buttocks. Move the person slowly and gently, being careful not to allow the person's body to bend or twist.

SPINAL DEFORMITIES

The two most common spinal deformities are scoliosis and kyphosis. Other spinal deformities that occur less frequently are spina bifida (below right) and spondylolisthesis (see page 127).

Kyphosis

Kyphosis is an abnormal degree of outward curvature of the spine. This condition usually affects the spine in the upper part of the back. Any degree of outward curvature of the spine in the lower back region or in the neck is abnormal. Kyphosis may be present at birth if the front portion of one or more vertebrae have not developed normally. Kyphosis that develops later in life is usually a result of spinal injury or disease but may also be caused by abnormal growth of the vertebrae. In some cases, kyphosis requires correction with a brace or by fusion of the vertebrae.

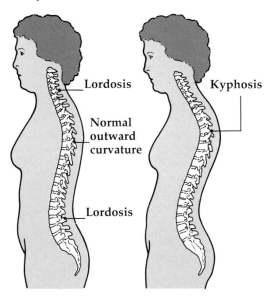

Normal and abnormal curves
Viewed from the side, a normal spine (above left) forms three curves – a lordosis (a curve that pushes inward at its apex) in the neck and another in the lower part of the back, and a curve that pushes outward in the upper part of the back. Kyphosis – an abnormal degree of outward curvature of the spine – in the upper part of the back (above right) is often caused by the bone disease osteoporosis.

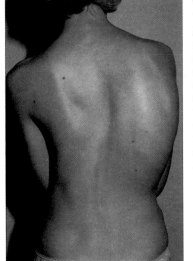

What causes scoliosis?
There are several types of scoliosis. Idiopathic scoliosis (shown at left) – the most common type – may begin in infancy, childhood, or adolescence. The cause of this type of scoliosis is unknown. In congenital scoliosis, a defect such as an abnormally developed vertebra is present at birth. Scoliosis develops rapidly as the child grows. Other causes of scoliosis include a difference in the length of the legs, a spinal tumor, arthritis or spasm of the back muscles on one side, or a neurological disorder affecting the back muscles.

Scoliosis

When viewed from the back, the normal spine forms a straight vertical line. In scoliosis, there is a sideways curvature and tilting of the spine.

Severe cases of scoliosis need treatment. A spinal brace and an exercise regimen may prevent further progression of the curvature. If this treatment is not successful, or if the curve is very severe, an operation to fuse the vertebrae may be performed. Severe scoliosis may damage the spinal cord, causing paralysis and interfering with breathing.

Spina bifida

About one in every 1,000 babies born has spina bifida, in which there is defective development of some of the vertebrae, with exposure of the spinal nerves, spinal cord, or the membranes covering the spinal cord. Spinal cord damage may develop as a result. Spina bifida most often occurs in the lower part of the back. The cause of the disorder is unknown; however, genetic (inherited) factors play a part. Symptoms can range from no handicap to severe physical handicap. The defect can be corrected surgically. Braces may aid mobility. In severe cases of spina bifida, many bodily systems, including the kidneys and lower part of the gastrointestinal tract, are affected.

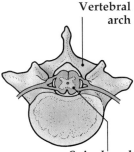

Normal spine

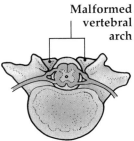

Spina bifida

A spinal defect at birth
The spinal cord is normally enclosed within arches of bone formed by the vertebrae (upper diagram). In some types of spina bifida, the spinal cord is incompletely enclosed by the vertebrae (lower diagram); this defect may result in damage to the spinal cord.

SURGICAL PROCEDURES
SPINAL FUSION

S PINAL FUSION **is an operation in
which adjacent vertebrae
in the spine are fused. This operation may be recommended for the
spinal instability caused by
spondylolisthesis, a condition in
which a vertebra slips forward
(see X-ray at right). Spinal fusion
may also be performed for unstable fractures of the spine or for
severe cases of spinal deformity.**

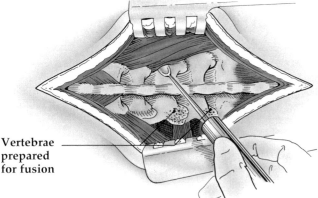

Spondylolisthesis
*This X-ray shows spondylolisthesis,
a condition in which a vertebra
(arrow) slips forward on another
vertebra. Mild cases of
spondylolisthesis may not cause
painful symptoms. Severe
spondylolisthesis may require an
operation, such as fusion of the two
vertebrae, to relieve pain.*

SPINAL FUSION FOR
SPONDYLOLISTHESIS

1 After administration of a general
anesthetic, the patient is positioned lying
face down on the operating table. The surgeon
makes an incision down the back. In some
cases, two incisions are made, one on either
side of the spine.

Incision

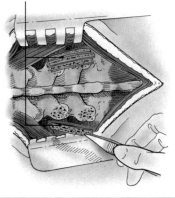

Vertebrae
prepared
for fusion

2 Through the incision, the surgeon lifts up
the muscles of the back to allow
access to the bony parts of the spine. He or
she identifies the slipped vertebra. The
slipped vertebra and the adjacent vertebra
are prepared for fusion by removing thin
slivers of bone from their sides.

Bone grafts

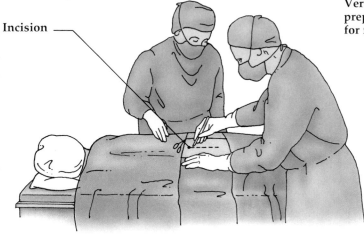

3 Bone for grafting is taken
from the back of the pelvis.
This bone is then laid on the
prepared sides of the vertebrae.
When the muscles are released,
they hold the grafts in position.
However, sometimes a fixation
device is used to provide
additional support. A drain is
usually inserted before the
incision is closed and is left in
place for 1 or 2 days to prevent
buildup of fluid.

4 Before being
allowed out of
bed, the patient may
be fitted with a brace
for back support.
When X-rays show
that the bones are
fusing satisfactorily,
usually after several
months, the brace can
be removed. The
patient can then start
a program of exercises
to strengthen the
muscles of the back
and abdomen.

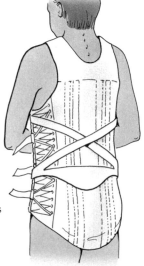

DRUGS FOR MUSCULOSKELETAL DISORDERS

Drug therapy plays an important part in the treatment of many disorders of the bones, muscles, and joints. Drugs may be prescribed to relieve pain and inflammation or to try to slow or stop the progression of an arthritic disease. New drugs are continuously being developed. This section will help you understand why your doctor has prescribed a drug, how to take the drug, how the drug works, and what side effects you may experience.

A variety of drugs are used to treat disorders of the musculoskeletal system, especially the inflammatory types of arthritis. Some drugs, such as nonsteroidal anti-inflammatory drugs (NSAIDs), are used to reduce inflammation and relieve symptoms. Other drugs, such as antirheumatics, are used to try to slow or stop progression of the underlying disease.

Drug groups
The majority of drugs that are used to treat musculoskeletal disorders can be grouped by how the drugs work or by the conditions the drugs are used to treat. Each of the drug groups listed above is reviewed in this section. For each group we de-

DRUG INDEX

If your doctor has prescribed a medication for you and you want to know more about the drug, the DRUG INDEX on page 139 will help you identify the group to which the drug belongs or the disorder for which the medication is usually prescribed.

scribe how the drugs work, why the drugs are prescribed, forms in which the drugs are taken, typical dosage frequencies, common side effects, and what to do if you miss a dose or if an overdose is taken. The most commonly prescribed drugs in each group are also listed. For some musculoskeletal disorders, your doctor may prescribe a combination of drugs. For example, treatment of rheumatoid arthritis may start with both NSAIDs and the slower-acting antirheumatic drugs.

USING PRESCRIPTION DRUGS SAFELY

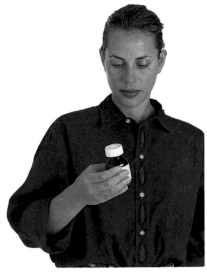

◆ Inform your doctor if there is a chance that you might be pregnant.

◆ Ask your doctor the name of the drug and what it is supposed to do. Be sure that you understand your doctor's instructions regarding the dosage of your medication.

◆ Take your medication as instructed. Do not take any more or less than the recommended dose.

◆ Always take the full treatment course of your medication. Do not stop taking medicine without talking to your doctor.

◆ Ask your doctor what foods, drinks, other drugs, or activities you should avoid while taking the drug.

◆ Call your doctor if you notice side effects or any change in the way a drug is affecting you.

◆ Store your medication under conditions (temperature and humidity) that ensure its effectiveness and keep it out of the reach of children.

◆ Ask your pharmacist to keep a complete list of your medications to monitor for drug interactions.

◆ Take a list of your prescription medications with you to doctors' appointments when consulting more than one doctor.

◆ Safely dispose of unused and outdated medications.

ANALGESIC DRUGS

Analgesic drugs are used to relieve pain. The most commonly used analgesic drugs are aspirin (which is also a nonsteroidal anti-inflammatory drug – see page 130) and acetaminophen. Narcotic drugs, such as codeine, are used only for short periods (a week or two) to treat severe pain.

How do they work?
Aspirin works by blocking the production of prostaglandins (pain-producing substances) throughout the body. Acetaminophen blocks the production of prostaglandins only in the brain. Narcotic analgesics produce their effect by imitating the action of natural pain-suppressing substances called endorphins that are formed in the brain to block the transmission of pain signals.

Who should not take analgesic drugs?
Aspirin or aspirin-containing preparations should never be given to children or teenagers unless recommended by your doctor, because these preparations have been linked to Reye's syndrome (degeneration of the liver and brain occurring after a viral infection).

You should not take aspirin if you are breast-feeding, if you take anticoagulant drugs, or if you have a peptic ulcer, gout, or hemophilia.

Consult your doctor before taking acetaminophen if you have liver or kidney problems.

How will the drugs affect me?
Analgesic drugs usually produce rapid relief from pain. Aspirin may cause abdominal pain, nausea, bleeding from the gastrointestinal tract, ringing in the ears, and allergic reactions. Side effects are common in people who need to take large doses. Acetaminophen is unlikely to produce side effects if taken at the dosage usually recommended.

ACTION OF ANALGESIC DRUGS
When body tissue is damaged, the body produces prostaglandins, which trigger the transmission of nerve signals that the brain interprets as pain. Analgesic drugs either block the production of prostaglandins (nonnarcotic analgesics) or interrupt the transmission of the pain signals (narcotic analgesics).

Action of narcotic analgesics
When body tissue is damaged (below left), prostaglandins are produced and trigger a pain signal that travels between nerve cells to the brain. Narcotic drugs block special pain receptors on brain cells (below center), preventing the transmission of the pain signal.

Action of nonnarcotics
Nonnarcotic analgesic drugs block the production of prostaglandins (below), preventing the stimulation of pain-sensitive nerve endings.

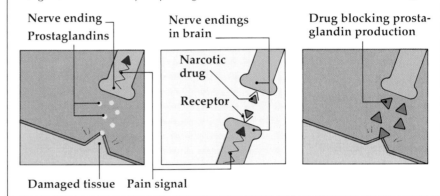

Nerve ending
Prostaglandins
Nerve endings in brain
Narcotic drug
Receptor
Drug blocking prostaglandin production
Damaged tissue   Pain signal

Possible side effects of narcotic analgesics include nausea, vomiting, constipation, and difficulty urinating. These drugs also cause drowsiness and may suppress breathing. Long-term use of narcotic analgesics causes addiction to the drugs.

How do I take the drugs?
Aspirin is usually taken after eating in the form of a coated tablet that does not dissolve in stomach acid; acetaminophen may be taken in tablet or syrup form. Aspirin and acetaminophen may be taken up to every 4 hours. Narcotic analgesics are usually taken by mouth; the dosage is determined by your doctor.

What happens if I miss a dose?
If you are no longer in pain, you do not need to take another dose of the analgesic. Otherwise, take the missed dose as soon as you can and don't take another dose for 4 hours.

Would an overdose be dangerous?
An overdose of aspirin can cause temporary hearing disturbances, mental confusion, abnormally deep or rapid breathing, and serious disturbances of metabolism. An acetaminophen overdose can cause liver damage. An overdose of a narcotic analgesic can be fatal.

How long will I have to take the drugs?
Analgesics are taken until the pain is relieved. In some cases, only one or two doses are needed.

COMMONLY USED ANALGESIC DRUGS
Nonnarcotic
Acetaminophen
Aspirin
Narcotic
Codeine
Propoxyphene

NSAIDs

Nonsteroidal anti-inflammatory drugs (NSAIDs), which include aspirin, are often used to relieve pain, stiffness, and inflammation in a wide variety of conditions affecting the bones, muscles, and joints, including rheumatoid arthritis (see page 84), osteoarthritis (see page 78), gout (see page 90), nonspecific back pain (see page 116), and muscle and tendon injuries (see page 102). These drugs are also used to treat systemic lupus erythematosus (see page 93) and pain caused by secondary bone tumors (see page 64).

Aspirin or another NSAID is often used during the initial phase of treatment of a musculoskeletal disorder or may be given when acetaminophen is ineffective or causes undesirable side effects. Your doctor may prescribe several different NSAIDs before finding the one that is most effective for you.

Drugs in the NSAID group are called "nonsteroidal" to distinguish them from corticosteroid drugs (see page 134), which have a more powerful anti-inflammatory effect but also may cause numerous and potentially serious side effects.

How do they work?

NSAIDs work by blocking the production of prostaglandins throughout the body – natural substances that cause pain and inflammation at the site of tissue damage.

Who should not take NSAIDs?

People who have peptic ulcers should avoid taking NSAIDs. If an NSAID is required in spite of a history of peptic ulcer, the stomach can be protected with other medications taken along with the NSAID. Elderly people; pregnant women; people with liver or kidney problems, allergic disorders, or bleeding disorders; and people taking anticoagulant drugs should talk to their doctor before taking an NSAID.

How will the drugs affect me?

In small doses, NSAIDs have an analgesic (painkilling) action, comparable to that of acetaminophen. In regular full dosages, NSAIDs have analgesic and anti-inflammatory actions, which makes NSAIDs useful for chronic painful or inflammatory conditions such as osteoarthritis and rheumatoid arthritis.

Most NSAIDs are effective in reducing inflammation, and thus reduce joint pain and swelling. When used regularly for prolonged periods, NSAIDs relieve stiffness and may improve joint function. NSAIDs will not, however, alter the progression of the underlying disease.

Common side effects include nausea, indigestion, bleeding from the stomach or upper part of the intestine, and diarrhea. Other side effects include allergic reactions, such as asthma and rashes, and kidney and liver damage. NSAIDs usually also impair the blood's ability to clot.

How do I take the drugs?

Most NSAIDs are taken by mouth. Oral NSAIDs should always be taken just after or with a meal to minimize the chance of stomach upset. Call your doctor if gastrointestinal or any other problems develop.

Most NSAIDs need to be taken three times a day to provide optimal pain relief. Some need to be taken

ACTION OF NSAIDs

NSAIDs are often prescribed to reduce the inflammation, pain, and stiffness that are caused by osteoarthritis. This disorder commonly affects weight-bearing joints, such as the hip joints (right). The cartilage lining the joint and covering the bones is damaged and triggers an inflammatory reaction in the tissues in the joint, causing pain and stiffness.

Synovial fluid

Healthy cartilage

Healthy joint tissues

Damaged cartilage

Inflamed joint tissues

Before the drug
In the joint disorder osteoarthritis, the protective layers of cartilage that line the joint and cover the bones are damaged and worn away; the tissues inside the joint are inflamed, causing stiffness and pain in the joint.

Drug

Reduced inflammation

After the drug
An NSAID reduces inflammation inside the joint, so the stiffness and pain are also reduced. NSAIDs do not enable the body to repair the damaged cartilage, so inflammation often recurs when you stop taking the drug.

only twice a day, and two (piroxicam and indomethacin) need to be taken only once a day. Treatment with most of the NSAIDs is started at a low dose and then increased to the dosage that produces maximum benefit without causing toxic effects.

What happens if I miss a dose?
If you forget to take a dose of an NSAID, take the missed dose as soon as you remember.

Would an overdose be dangerous?
A single extra dose of an NSAID is unlikely to have a serious adverse effect, but there is a danger of bleeding in the stomach or duodenum (part of the small intestine). Call your doctor if a large overdose is taken.

How long will I have to take the drugs?
The length of your treatment with an NSAID depends on the disease or disorder. Some muscle or tendon injuries need only a short course of treatment. You may need to take NSAIDs for longer periods (sometimes indefinitely) if you have a chronic form of arthritis.

COMMONLY USED NSAIDs
Aspirin
Diclofenac
Diflunisal
Fenoprofen
Flurbiprofen
Ibuprofen
Indomethacin
Ketoprofen
Meclofenamate
Mefenamic acid
Naproxen
Phenylbutazone
Piroxicam
Salsalate
Sodium salicylate
Sulindac
Tolmetin

ANTIRHEUMATIC DRUGS

Antirheumatic drugs are used to treat people with rheumatoid arthritis whose symptoms are not relieved by NSAIDs (see page 130).

Antirheumatic drugs are prescribed to slow or stop progression of the underlying arthritic disease. These drugs include gold derivatives, penicillamine, antimalarial drugs, sulfasalazine, and immunosuppressant drugs.

How do they work?
The action of some antirheumatic drugs (penicillamine and gold derivatives) is not fully understood. Immunosuppressant drugs suppress the body's immune responses (believed to be partly responsible for rheumatoid arthritis).

Who should not take antirheumatic drugs?
Almost all types of antirheumatic drugs are not prescribed for people who have blood disorders, pulmonary fibrosis (extensive scarring of the lungs), or severe kidney or liver disease. These drugs are not usually prescribed for pregnant women.

How will the drugs affect me?
Antirheumatic drugs may prevent further damage to cartilage and bone, slowing the progression of joint deformity, reducing pain and disability, and increasing mobility. The intended beneficial effects may take weeks or months to appear.

Side effects of antirheumatic drugs may be severe. Gold derivatives, penicillamine, sulfasalazine, and immunosuppressants all have the potential for causing life-threatening complications. Your doctor will closely supervise your treatment. The antimalarial drugs chloroquine and hydroxychloroquine may cause damage to the retina, so you should see your ophthalmologist regularly.

ACTION OF ANTIRHEUMATIC DRUGS

Antirheumatic drugs are often prescribed to treat rheumatoid arthritis, a condition that most commonly affects the joints of the hands and fingers (below). The joints become swollen and painful and may become deformed.

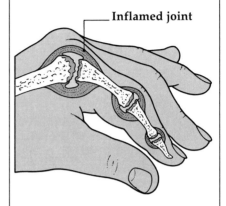

Inflamed joint

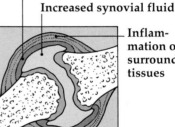

Inflamed synovial membrane

Increased synovial fluid

Inflammation of surrounding tissues

Before the drug
In a joint affected by acute rheumatoid arthritis, the synovial membrane is inflamed and excess synovial fluid is produced, causing pain and stiffness. The tissues surrounding the affected joint also become inflamed.

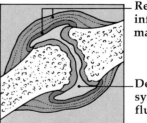

Reduced inflammation

Decreased synovial fluid

After the drug
Treatment with an antirheumatic drug may prevent progression of rheumatoid arthritis. Inflammation is reduced.

How do I take the drugs?

Gold derivatives are either taken daily by mouth or given by injection. Penicillamine tablets are taken daily before eating. Chloroquine and hydroxychloroquine tablets are usually taken daily after eating. Sulfasalazine is taken orally four times a day after eating. Immunosuppressants are taken orally once or twice a day. Methotrexate is taken orally once a week.

What happens if I miss a dose?

If you forget to take a dose of an antirheumatic drug, omit the missed dose and take the next dose at its regularly scheduled time.

Would an overdose be dangerous?

A single extra dose of an antirheumatic drug is unlikely to have a serious adverse effect; call your doctor if a large overdose is taken.

How long will I have to take the drugs?

Treatment with gold derivatives, sulfasalazine, and penicillamine may need to be continued for months or until remission of the disease occurs. Immunosuppressant drugs and chloroquine are not usually taken for longer than 2 years because of possible adverse effects.

COMMONLY USED
ANTIRHEUMATIC DRUGS
Gold derivatives
Auranofin
Aurothioglucose
Immunosuppressants
Azathioprine
Chlorambucil
Cyclophosphamide
Methotrexate
Other drugs
Chloroquine
Hydroxychloroquine
Penicillamine
Sulfasalazine

DRUGS FOR GOUT

Drugs prescribed to treat gout (see page 90) can be divided into two categories – those used to treat acute attacks and those used to prevent recurrent attacks.

Acute attacks of gout are usually treated with NSAIDs (see page 130) or colchicine. Corticotropin or a corticosteroid drug (see page 134) is sometimes used for a short time. If you are susceptible to recurrent attacks of gout, you should always carry your medication with you so that you can take it immediately when another attack begins.

Allopurinol, probenecid, or sulfinpyrazone may be prescribed to help prevent attacks of gout.

How do they work?

The way in which colchicine works is not known. Corticotropin, corticosteroids, and NSAIDs work by reducing the inflammatory response in affected joints.

Allopurinol reduces the level of uric acid in the blood by interfering with the activity of an enzyme involved in uric acid production. Probenecid and sulfinpyrazone work by increasing the amount of uric acid that is excreted in the urine.

Who should not take drugs for gout?

Probenecid and sulfinpyrazone are not usually prescribed for people who excrete excessive amounts of uric acid in their urine because these

---

ACTION OF DRUGS FOR GOUT

The kidneys remove excess uric acid from the body by filtering the uric acid from the blood and excreting it in the urine. Excessive levels of uric acid may occur in the blood if too much uric acid is being produced by the body or if kidney function is impaired. If the crystals of uric acid accumulate in a joint (most commonly the big toe or knee or the joints of the hand), they can cause attacks of gout. In people with high levels of uric acid in the blood, these levels can be reduced by treatment with drugs that increase the amount of uric acid excreted by the kidneys.

How the kidney filters blood
The illustration at right shows a kidney and an enlarged view of one of its filtering units – called a nephron. The nephrons consist of a glomerulus and a tubule. The glomerulus removes waste products (such as uric acid) and water from the bloodstream; the water and waste products then pass down the tubule. Some of the water is reabsorbed into the bloodstream; the waste products and the remaining water are excreted as urine via the ureter.

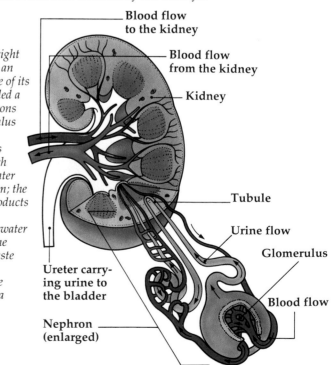

Blood flow to the kidney

Blood flow from the kidney

Kidney

Tubule

Urine flow

Glomerulus

Blood flow

Ureter carrying urine to the bladder

Nephron (enlarged)

drugs further increase the output of uric acid and increase the risk of stone formation in the kidneys.

Treatment with allopurinol, probenecid, and sulfinpyrazone should not be started during an acute attack of gout, because these drugs could worsen the attack.

How will the drugs affect me?

NSAIDs and colchicine ease symptoms of an acute attack if the medication is taken as soon as the attack begins. Corticotropin or a corticosteroid may be prescribed if an NSAID or colchicine is not successful.

The most common side effects of colchicine are nausea, vomiting, diarrhea, and abdominal pain. The side effects of NSAIDs are described on page 130. Corticotropin or a corticosteroid is unlikely to cause any adverse effects over the brief time that either drug is used.

Allopurinol, probenecid, and sulfinpyrazone are usually successful in preventing attacks of gout and the subsequent joint deformity.

How do I take the drugs?

Colchicine and NSAIDs are taken by mouth four times a day. A corticosteroid drug may be prescribed to be taken orally for several days in gradually decreasing dosages. Corticotropin is given by intramuscular injection. Allopurinol, probenecid, and sulfinpyrazone are taken orally one to four times a day.

Attacks of gout may be triggered by starting preventive treatment with allopurinol, probenecid, or sulfinpyrazone, so colchicine or an NSAID is usually also given with the first few months' treatment.

You should always drink plenty of fluids while you are taking preventive medication for gout.

What happens if I miss a dose?

A single missed dose is unlikely to have a serious adverse effect, but symptoms may recur. Take the missed dose as soon as you can. If the next dose is due within an hour or so, omit the missed dose.

Would an overdose be dangerous?

Call your doctor if you take an overdose of colchicine. If nausea, vomiting, bloody diarrhea, or severe abdominal pain occurs, go to the nearest hospital emergency room; some adverse reactions can be fatal.

A single extra dose of allopurinol, probenecid, or sulfinpyrazone is unlikely to be serious, but call your doctor if an overdose is taken.

How long will I have to take the drugs?

NSAIDs, colchicine, and corticosteroids are usually taken for only a few days, until symptoms subside. A single injection of corticotropin is usually sufficient. Treatment with allopurinol, probenecid, or sulfinpyrazone continues indefinitely.

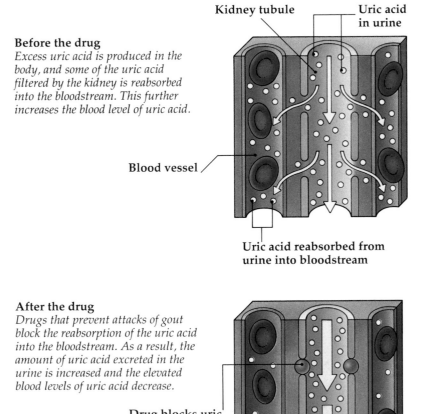

Before the drug
Excess uric acid is produced in the body, and some of the uric acid filtered by the kidney is reabsorbed into the bloodstream. This further increases the blood level of uric acid.

Kidney tubule

Uric acid in urine

Blood vessel

Uric acid reabsorbed from urine into bloodstream

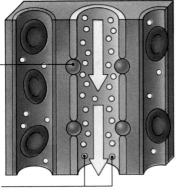

After the drug
Drugs that prevent attacks of gout block the reabsorption of the uric acid into the bloodstream. As a result, the amount of uric acid excreted in the urine is increased and the elevated blood levels of uric acid decrease.

Drug blocks uric acid reabsorption

Increased uric acid excreted in urine

COMMONLY USED
DRUGS FOR GOUT
Allopurinol
Colchicine
Corticosteroids
Corticotropin
NSAIDs
Prednisone
Probenecid
Sulfinpyrazone
Triamcinolone

CORTICOSTEROID DRUGS

Corticosteroids are hormones produced by the adrenal glands. These hormones play an important role in inhibiting the body's immune system and in regulating the metabolism of carbohydrates and minerals.

Corticosteroid drugs, which are either identical to or closely related to corticosteroid hormones, may be prescribed to treat some joint disorders when treatment with other types of anti-inflammatory drugs has been unsuccessful in relieving pain and swelling. When corticosteroid drugs are used to treat complications of osteoarthritis (see page 78), bursitis (see page 100), or gout (see page 90), the injectable form of the drug is used. Corticosteroid drugs may also be prescribed to relieve inflammation of soft tissues around joints.

Corticosteroid drugs (in small doses) are also used to treat polymyalgia rheumatica and temporal arteritis (see page 113), systemic lupus erythematosus (see page 93), and polymyositis (see page 112).

How do they work?

Corticosteroids inhibit the activity of white blood cells. They also block the production of prostaglandins, substances that trigger pain and inflammation in the affected area.

Who should not take corticosteroid drugs?

When possible, long-term treatment with corticosteroids is avoided in children, because the drugs may stunt growth. Corticosteroids are not usually prescribed for people with peptic ulcers or people who have, or are at risk of, serious infection.

How will the drugs affect me?

Corticosteroid drugs injected into an inflamed joint reduce the inflammatory response (pain and swelling) in the joint. A limited number of corticosteroid injections is unlikely to have serious adverse effects.

Long-term treatment with oral corticosteroid drugs can cause hypertension (high blood pressure), demineralization of bone and fractures, peptic ulcers, diabetes mellitus, muscle weakness, swelling of the face and other parts of the body, acne, cataracts, and excessive growth of facial hair in women. Your doctor will closely supervise your drug treatment to monitor your condition for adverse effects.

ACTION OF CORTICOSTEROID DRUGS

Corticosteroids may be injected into particularly painful joints that have become damaged by osteoarthritis or rheumatoid arthritis. The joints most commonly treated with corticosteroid injections are the knees, shoulders, and fingers. In some cases, corticosteroids may be injected into other joints to relieve severe pain caused by conditions such as inflammation of the synovial membrane or the joint capsule.

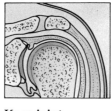
Shoulder joint

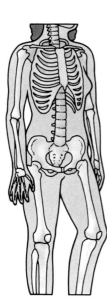

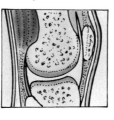
Knee joint

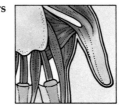
Fingers

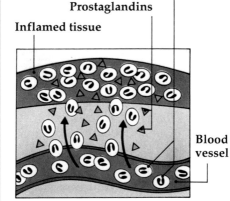

White blood cells

Prostaglandins

Inflamed tissue

Blood vessel

Before the drug
When tissues are damaged, substances called prostaglandins are released and cause large numbers of white blood cells and fluid to accumulate in the damaged tissue. The result is an inflammatory response consisting of pain and swelling.

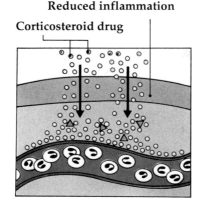

Reduced inflammation

Corticosteroid drug

After the drug
When a corticosteroid drug is injected into the affected area, the drug enters the synovial membrane that lines the joint and reduces the inflammatory response in the damaged tissue, in part by blocking the production of prostaglandins. Pain is relieved and swelling is reduced.

How do I take the drugs?

Oral corticosteroids, taken daily or on alternate days, may be prescribed to treat generalized disorders.

For some of the localized disorders or injuries, a corticosteroid drug may be given by injection directly into the affected area.

What happens if I miss a dose?

You should take the missed dose as soon as you remember. If the next dose is due in an hour or so, omit the missed dose. You should never stop taking oral corticosteroids without consulting your doctor; serious side effects may occur.

Would an overdose be dangerous?

An extra dose is unlikely to have any serious effects. Call your doctor if you have taken a large overdose.

How long will I have to take the drugs?

In most cases, a single injection of a corticosteroid drug usually relieves pain and swelling and improves mobility. Occasionally, repeated injections (limited to no more than four in 1 year) are given.

Treatment with oral corticosteroids may need to continue as long as is necessary to control the disease. For example, treatment of polymyalgia rheumatica can continue for as long as 3 years or more.

When treatment with oral corticosteroids is stopped, the dosage must be reduced gradually. Serious, life-threatening adverse reactions may occur if the drug treatment is stopped abruptly.

COMMONLY USED
CORTICOSTEROID DRUGS
Hydrocortisone
Methylprednisolone
Prednisolone
Prednisone
Triamcinolone

MUSCLE RELAXANTS

Muscle relaxants are primarily used to treat muscle spasticity caused by certain neuromuscular disorders. These drugs are also sometimes prescribed for short periods to treat severe, painful muscle spasms resulting from an injury (see page 102) or occasionally from osteoarthritis (see page 78). The effects of muscle relaxants in the treatment of osteoarthritis are unpredictable and of questionable value; muscle spasms that may occur with osteoarthritis are often relieved when pain is controlled.

How do they work?

Most muscle relaxants act on the central nervous system (the brain and spinal cord). They block receptors on the nerve cells that are used by neurotransmitters to transmit signals to the muscles. The suppressed stimulation reduces muscle contraction and relaxes spastic muscles. Dantrolene acts on skeletal muscles, reducing their sensitivity to nerve signals.

Who should not take muscle relaxants?

People with peptic ulcers should not take baclofen; dantrolene should not be taken by children.

How will the drugs affect me?

Muscle relaxants may reduce stiffness and improve mobility in people with severe muscle spasms. Relaxation of the spasms often enables physical therapy to be carried out more effectively.

Most muscle relaxants have a depressant effect on the body's nervous system and cause drowsiness. Dependence may develop with long-term use of muscle relaxants. If the drug treatment is stopped suddenly, muscle stiffness may worsen.

ACTION OF MUSCLE RELAXANTS

Muscle movements are the result of signals that originate in the brain and pass down the spinal cord and along the nerves to the muscle. Muscle spasms are involuntary, prolonged, painful contractions of a muscle caused by excessive stimulation of the muscle. Muscle relaxants that act on the central nervous system slow down the passage of the signals to the muscles.

Before the drug
The neurotransmitters in the central nervous system transmit an excessive number of signals to a muscle, overstimulating the muscle and causing spasms.

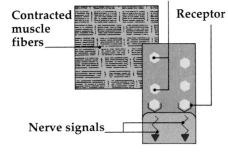

Neurotransmitters

Receptor

Contracted muscle fibers

Nerve signals

Relaxed muscle fibers

Drug occupying receptor

Nerve signal

After the drug
Muscle relaxants that act on the central nervous system occupy some of the receptor sites on the nerve cells that normally transmit the signals. As a result, fewer signals can reach the spastic muscle, allowing the muscle fibers to relax.

Dantrolene can cause liver damage, so periodic blood tests are needed to monitor your liver function.

How do I take the drugs?
Diazepam is taken orally four times a day. In cases of acute muscle spasms, your doctor may inject diazepam. Baclofen is taken by mouth a few times a day, preferably after eating. Dantrolene is taken by mouth one or more times a day.

Your doctor may have to adjust the dosage of a muscle relaxant in order to find the most appropriate dosage that controls your symptoms yet maintains sufficient strength of your muscles.

What happens if I miss a dose?
A single missed dose generally does not cause any serious adverse effects. You should take the missed dose as soon as you remember. If the next dose is due in an hour or so, omit the missed dose.

Would an overdose be dangerous?
An overdose of a muscle relaxant causes profound drowsiness and muscle weakness. Call your doctor immediately if you have taken a large overdose of a muscle relaxant.

How long will I have to take the drugs?
Muscle relaxants may have to be taken indefinitely for chronic neuromuscular conditions associated with muscle spasms. These drugs produce sufficient relaxation of spastic muscles to allow a person with such a condition to have a limited degree of flexibility and mobility.

COMMONLY USED
MUSCLE RELAXANTS
Baclofen
Cyclobenzaprine
Dantrolene
Diazepam

DRUGS FOR BONE DISORDERS

A number of drugs are used to treat bone disorders, such as osteomalacia and rickets (see page 60), osteoporosis (see page 58), and Paget's disease (see page 62). In some cases, treatment may include a combination of drugs.

Calcitonin and etidronate are used mainly in the treatment of Paget's disease. Vitamin D is used to treat osteomalacia and rickets.

Estrogen therapy can help reduce the risk or progression of osteoporosis in postmenopausal women.

Calcium carbonate may be used as a dietary calcium supplement for people with osteomalacia, rickets, and osteoporosis.

How do they work?
The drugs used to treat bone disorders have different effects on bone protein and minerals.

Calcitonin, along with parathyroid hormone, helps regulate the metabolism of bone to prevent abnormal bone formation. Etidronate reduces the rate of bone formation and breakdown.

Vitamin D enhances the absorption of calcium from the intestinal

ACTION OF DRUGS FOR BONE DISORDERS

Normal, healthy bone has a hard, strong, external structure and a softer, central core that contains the bone marrow. Bone cells, regulated by hormones, take nutrients from the blood and use them in a process of constant rebuilding (called remodeling) of the hard, mineralized bone tissue.

Strong bone structure

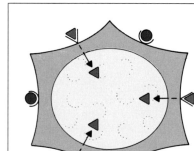

Minerals used by bone   **Natural hormones**

Healthy bone
Bone with normal mineral density has balanced levels of hormonal activity and mineral supply.

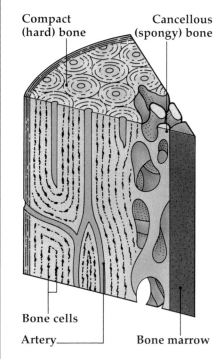

Compact (hard) bone   **Cancellous (spongy) bone**

Bone cells

Artery   **Bone marrow**

Compact bone
Each main bone of the body has a significant proportion of compact (cortical) bone, which gives the bone its hardness and strength. Compact bone is formed by the action of millions of bone cells; if the normal activities of these cells are disturbed through lack of vitamins, minerals, or hormones, the bones may weaken.

tract and is essential for normal growth of strong, healthy bones.

Estrogen therapy, if started with the onset of menopause and taken over a long period, can reduce post-menopausal loss of bone. Calcium carbonate may also help maintain the mineral content of bone.

Who should not take drugs for bone disorders?

Estrogen should not be taken during pregnancy or by women with a history of uterine cancer, hypertension (high blood pressure), thrombosis (formation of a blood clot in a blood vessel), or impaired liver function.

How will the drugs affect me?

Calcitonin and etidronate relieve pain and stimulate bone growth in Paget's disease and may also be used in the treatment of osteoporosis. Both of these drugs may cause gastro-intestinal disturbances and alter-ations in your sense of taste.

Treatment with vitamin D may restore strength to softened bones in people with osteomalacia.

Treatment with estrogen does not strengthen bones weakened by osteoporosis but may help to pre-vent further weakening. Possible side effects of estrogen include spot-ting of blood from the vagina, nau-sea, vomiting, weight gain, and headache. Estrogen taken without progesterone requires periodic ex-amination of the lining of the uterus.

How do I take the drugs?

Calcitonin is given in the form of an injection usually three times a week. Etidronate is usually taken daily by mouth between meals. Vitamin D is usually taken daily by mouth. Estro-gen is usually taken by mouth, usu-ally in combination with progester-one, for 21 days each month. Cal-cium carbonate is taken orally, one to four times a day.

What happens if I miss a dose?

Missing a dose of any of these drugs for bone disorders is unlikely to have a serious adverse effect. Take the missed dose as soon as you can.

Would an overdose be dangerous?

An extra dose is unlikely to have any serious adverse effects. However, too much calcium or vitamin D can cause abnormally high levels of calcium in the blood. If you are taking high doses of vitamin D regularly, you should have your blood level of calcium checked periodically. Symptoms of overdosage include loss of appetite, tiredness, gastrointestinal distur-bances, weight loss, headache, and excessive thirst.

How long will I have to take the drugs?

Drugs for bone disorders may have to be taken for many months or even years until symptoms resolve.

> COMMONLY USED DRUGS
> FOR BONE DISORDERS
> Calcitonin
> Calcium carbonate
> Estrogens
> Etidronate
> Vitamin D

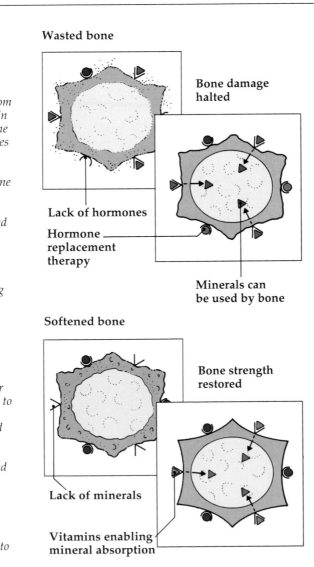

Bone damaged by osteoporosis
Lack of hormones has prevented bone cells from utilizing the minerals in the blood to rebuild bone tissue, causing the bones to become fragile and brittle (osteoporosis). Treatment with hormone and mineral supple-ments, along with appropriate exercise and avoiding those things that contribute to osteoporosis (see page 59), helps prevent the bone from degenerating further but cannot restore lost bone mass.

Bone damaged by osteomalacia
In osteomalacia, deficiency of calcium or vitamin D causes bone to soften. As a result, the bones become weak and can eventually become deformed. Drug treat-ment with vitamins and minerals, along with treatment of any gastro-intestinal cause of the deficiency, generally restores bone strength to normal levels.

Wasted bone

Bone damage halted

Lack of hormones

Hormone replacement therapy

Minerals can be used by bone

Softened bone

Bone strength restored

Lack of minerals

Vitamins enabling mineral absorption

DRUGS FOR MYASTHENIA GRAVIS

Neostigmine and pyridostigmine are the drugs most often used to improve muscle function in myasthenia gravis (see page 111). These drugs may be used alone or with other drugs, such as corticosteroids or azathioprine, that suppress the body's immune system.

How do they work?

Muscles contract in response to a substance called acetylcholine, which is released from nerve fibers to stimulate receptors on muscle cells. Neostigmine and pyridostigmine block the action of the enzyme that destroys acetylcholine. These drugs thus increase the amount of acetylcholine that is available and so prolong the response of muscle cells to stimulation by nerve signals.

Who should not take drugs for myasthenia gravis?

Neostigmine and pyridostigmine should not be taken by people who have narrowing of the urinary or intestinal tracts.

How will the drugs affect me?

The drugs have no effect on the disease process itself but usually restore muscle function to a normal or near-normal level, particularly in mild cases. These drugs can produce unwanted muscular activity by enhancing the transmission of nerve impulses elsewhere in the body.

Common side effects include nausea, vomiting, diarrhea, increased perspiration, and muscle and intestinal cramps.

Corticosteroid drugs begin to relieve symptoms after about 2 weeks. These drugs may be taken daily or on alternate days.

How do I take the drugs?

The drugs are taken a few times a day, by mouth or as an injection.

ACTION OF DRUGS FOR MYASTHENIA GRAVIS

In myasthenia gravis, certain antibodies produced in the thymus gland disrupt nerve signals between the nervous system and some of the muscles. As a result, the affected muscles become progressively weaker. The muscles first affected are usually those of the face (particularly the eyelids), larynx (voice box), and pharynx (back of the throat); as the disease progresses, the muscles of the arms (especially the shoulders) and legs also become affected.

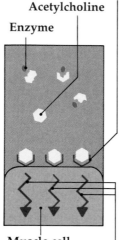
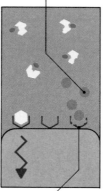
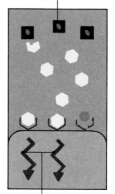

Normal muscle activity
When you want to move a muscle, a nerve signal is sent to the muscle. Acetylcholine (released from nerve fibers) binds to receptors on muscle cells and transmits the signal, causing the muscle to contract. An enzyme breaks down excess acetylcholine.

Muscle action in myasthenia gravis
In myasthenia gravis, antibodies produced by the thymus gland destroy many of the receptors on the muscle cells. Fewer muscle receptors are available for the acetylcholine to bind to, so the resulting signal that causes the muscle to contract is weak.

After the drug
The drug blocks the action of the enzyme that normally breaks down acetylcholine. More acetylcholine is therefore available to stimulate the reduced number of receptors on the muscle cells, and the muscle response to the nerve signals is increased.

What happens if I miss a dose?

Symptoms are likely to return if a dose of neostigmine or pyridostigmine is missed. Take the missed dose as soon as you remember. If the next dose is due in an hour or so, omit the missed dose.

Would an overdose be dangerous?

Large overdoses of neostigmine or pyridostigmine can cause further muscle weakness. Call your doctor if you have taken an overdose.

How long will I have to take the drugs?

Unless the condition can be successfully treated by surgery (total or partial removal of the thymus gland), these drugs may have to be taken indefinitely. Your doctor will monitor your treatment for side effects.

> **COMMONLY USED DRUGS FOR MYASTHENIA GRAVIS**
> Corticosteroids
> Neostigmine
> Pyridostigmine

DRUG INDEX

How to use the index

All entries in this index are generic names (recognized medical names) of drugs used to treat or prevent disorders affecting the bones, muscles, or joints. Most entries cross-refer you to one of the drug groups on pages 129 through 138. Brand names of drugs are not included in this index. If your doctor has prescribed a brand-name product, you can generally determine the generic name by asking your doctor or pharmacist or by reading the package insert.

A

acetaminophen a nonnarcotic analgesic (painkiller)

allopurinol a drug used to prevent attacks of gout

aspirin an NSAID

auranofin an antirheumatic gold compound

aurothioglucose an antirheumatic gold compound

azathioprine an immunosuppressant also used as an antirheumatic

B-C

baclofen a muscle relaxant

calcitonin a hormone drug used to treat bone disorders

calcium carbonate a drug used to treat bone disorders

chlorambucil an anticancer drug also used as an antirheumatic

chloroquine an antimalarial also used as an antirheumatic

codeine a narcotic analgesic (painkiller)

colchicine a drug used to treat and prevent attacks of gout

corticotropin a hormone drug used to treat attacks of gout

cyclobenzaprine a muscle relaxant

cyclophosphamide an anticancer drug also used as an antirheumatic

D-F

dantrolene a muscle relaxant

diazepam a muscle relaxant; also used to treat anxiety

diclofenac an NSAID

diflunisal an NSAID

estrogens hormone drugs used as hormone replacement therapy, which helps reduce the risk of the bone disorder osteoporosis in postmenopausal women (decreased bone mineral density)

etidronate a drug used to treat Paget's disease (a bone formation disorder in middle-aged and older people) and osteoporosis (decreased bone mineral density)

fenoprofen an NSAID

flurbiprofen an NSAID

H

hydrocortisone a corticosteroid

hydroxychloroquine an antimalarial also used as an antirheumatic

I-K

ibuprofen an NSAID

indomethacin an NSAID

ketoprofen an NSAID

M

magnesium salicylate used as an analgesic (painkiller) anti-inflammatory to treat arthritis

meclofenamate an NSAID

mefenamic acid an NSAID

methotrexate an anticancer drug also used as an antirheumatic

methylprednisolone a corticosteroid

morphine a narcotic analgesic (painkiller)

N-P

naproxen an NSAID

neostigmine a drug used to treat myasthenia gravis (muscle disorder)

penicillamine an antirheumatic

phenylbutazone an NSAID

piroxicam an NSAID

prednisolone a corticosteroid

prednisone a corticosteroid

probenecid a drug used to increase urinary excretion of uric acid and thus reduce blood levels of uric acid that occur with gout

propoxyphene a narcotic analgesic (painkiller)

pyridostigmine a drug used to treat myasthenia gravis (muscle disorder)

S

salsalate an NSAID

sodium salicylate an NSAID

sulfasalazine an antibacterial and anti-inflammatory also used as an antirheumatic

sulfinpyrazone a drug used to increase urinary excretion of uric acid and thus reduce blood levels of uric acid that occur with gout

sulindac an NSAID

T-V

tolmetin an NSAID

triamcinolone a corticosteroid

vitamin D a vitamin used to treat some bone disorders

GLOSSARY OF TERMS AND DISORDERS

Words in *italics* refer to other definitions included in this glossary. All of the musculoskeletal disorders included in this volume are not listed in this glossary. Please refer to the index on pages 142 to 144.

A

Abduction
Movement of a limb away from the central plane of the body, or movement of a digit away from the long axis of a limb. Abduction is the opposite of *adduction*.

Achilles tendon
The thick, strong tendon formed from muscles in the calf and attached to the heel bone (calcaneus).

Achondroplasia
A genetic disorder of bone growth in which the cartilage at the end of the long bones does not develop normally, resulting in stunted growth (called dwarfism) and abnormal body proportions.

Adduction
Movement of a limb toward the central plane of the body, or movement of a digit toward the long axis of a limb. Adduction is the opposite of *abduction*.

Ankylosis
Complete immobility of a joint that results from disease or injury or from a surgical procedure that fuses a joint (called *arthrodesis*).

Arthrodesis
A surgical procedure in which a severely damaged or deformed joint is fused to prevent bone movement, relieving pain and improving stability of the joint.

Arthropathy
Any disease or disorder that affects the joints.

Arthroplasty
The surgical replacement of a joint by artificial components.

B - C

Bone cyst
An abnormal bone cavity, usually filled with fluid. Cysts can weaken bone, increasing the risk of fracture.

Carpal tunnel syndrome
A condition characterized by numbness, tingling, and pain in the hand, especially at night, caused by pressure on the median nerve as it passes between the bones and a ligament at the front of the wrist. Supporting the wrist in a splint and injecting the wrist with a corticosteroid drug may alleviate symptoms. Surgery is needed in some cases.

Cervical osteoarthritis
Degeneration of the joints between vertebrae in the neck, causing neck pain and stiffness. The diagnosis is confirmed by X-ray, and treatment includes painkilling drugs and physical therapy.

Cervical rib syndrome
A condition characterized by pain, numbness, and tingling in the arm and hand caused by an extra rib in the neck that presses on the nerves and blood vessels. Physical therapy may relieve symptoms. Surgery is needed in some cases.

Chondritis
Inflammation of cartilage.

Chondroma
A benign tumor of cartilage cells that develops either on the surface of cartilage (ecchondroma) or inside bone or cartilage (enchondroma). Many chondromas do not require treatment.

Chondromalacia patellae
Painful degeneration of the cartilage behind the kneecap (patella) that most commonly affects adolescents. Treatment includes supporting and resting the knee, strengthening the thigh (quadriceps) muscle, and taking anti-inflammatory medication.

Compartmental syndrome
Painful compression of a group of muscles that results in a reduced blood supply to the muscles, most often caused by injury or excessive exercise.

Coxa vara
A hip deformity in which the angle formed between the neck of the femur and the shaft of the femur is reduced, causing shortening of the leg. Surgery may be needed.

Cramp
Brief, painful, strong contraction of a muscle.

D

Dermatomyositis
A connective-tissue disorder that causes muscle weakness and rash. Treatment may include corticosteroids and immunosuppressants.

Dupuytren's contracture
Thickening and tightening of the tissues in the palm of the hand, causing the fourth and fifth fingers to become fixed in a bent position. Surgery may be needed in severe cases.

E

Ehlers-Danlos syndrome
A disorder affecting collagen (a structural protein), characterized by abnormal stretchiness of skin, poor wound healing, easy bruising, joint instability, and skeletal abnormalities.

Ewing's tumor
A rare cancer of the bone that most commonly occurs in children. The tumor develops in bone marrow, usually of a long bone in an arm or leg. Treatment may include radiation therapy and chemotherapy (anticancer drugs).

Exostosis
A benign bone tumor that projects from the surface of the affected bone. The growth may be removed surgically if necessary.

Extension
A movement in which two adjoining bones are straightened. The opposite is *flexion*.

F

Fibrosarcoma
A rare cancer of connective tissue that may develop in bone or around a muscle or tendon. Treatment may include surgical removal, chemotherapy (anticancer drugs), and radiation therapy.

Flexion
A movement in which two adjoining bones are bent. The opposite is *extension*.

Frozen shoulder
Pain, stiffness, and limitation of movement in the shoulder joint caused by inflammation and thickening of the *joint capsule*. Treatment includes NSAIDs such as aspirin, physical therapy, and, occasionally, manipulation of the shoulder with the use of an anesthetic.

G - H

Ganglion
A fluid-filled swelling, associated with a tendon sheath or *joint capsule*, most commonly occurring at the back of the wrist. Treatment, when needed, consists of removal of the fluid through a needle and injection of a corticosteroid drug or surgical removal of the ganglion.

Hallux rigidus
Pain and loss of movement at the base of the big toe due to osteoarthritis. Surgery may be needed in severe cases.

Hammer toe
A deformity of the toe in which the main toe joint is bent upward. A protective pad may help relieve pain. Surgery may be needed in severe cases.

Hemarthrosis
Bleeding into a joint cavity, usually resulting from injury. Less commonly, hemarthrosis results from a bleeding disorder, such as hemophilia.

Hyperuricemia
An abnormally high level of uric acid in the blood, which may lead to gout.

J

Joint capsule
The tough, fibrous tissue that encloses a joint.

Joint effusion
Accumulation of fluid inside a joint, usually resulting from injury or inflammation. Treatment may include the removal of the fluid from the joint through a needle, resting the affected joint, antibiotics, and applying ice.

K - L

Kyphosis
Excessive outward curvature of the spine, usually in the upper part of the back.

Lordosis
The inward curvature of the spine in the neck and in the lower part of the back.

Lumbago
Pain in the lower part of the back, usually caused by disc prolapse (rupture), arthritis, or muscle or ligament strain. Treatment usually includes bed rest or wearing a brace.

M

March fracture
A fracture of a metatarsal bone in the foot, also called metatarsal stress fracture, usually caused by running or walking long distances on hard surfaces. Treatment is usually to rest the foot, sometimes by immobilization in a cast.

Meniscus
A crescent-shaped disc of cartilage found in some joints.

Metatarsalgia
Pain in the top of the foot, usually caused by a lack of arch in the foot, a *march fracture*, or pinching of a nerve in the foot.

Myositis
Painful inflammation of muscle, which may be caused by infection, injury, or a disorder of the body's immune system.

N - O

Neuropathic joint
A joint that has become progessively damaged as a result of a nerve disorder that has caused a loss of sensation in the joint.

Orthopedics
The branch of medicine concerned with the diagnosis and treatment of diseases of the musculoskeletal system.

Osgood-Schlatter disease
Painful enlargement of the bony prominence just below the knee, most commonly occurring in adolescent boys, caused by strain at the point of attachment of the patellar tendon. Treatment is not usually needed.

Ossification
The process of bone formation.

Osteitis pubis
Painful inflammation of the joint in the front of the pelvis where the two pubic bones join. It is common in women. Treatment may include bed rest, NSAIDs such as aspirin, and physical therapy.

Osteochondritis dissecans
Separation of a segment of bone just under a joint surface, usually within the knee or ankle. The disorder usually starts in adolescence and causes pain and stiffness. Treatment is generally to rest the affected joint. Surgery may be needed in some cases.

Osteoma
A benign bone tumor that may occur on any bone, forming a rounded swelling. Surgery may be needed in some cases.

Osteopetrosis
A rare inherited disorder in which bone becomes abnormally dense.

Osteophytes
Outgrowths of bone that develop at the edges of joints that are affected by the bone disease osteoarthritis.

Osteotomy
An operation in which a bone is cut or fractured in order to change the length of the bone, to correct deformity, or to improve stability of a joint.

P

Painful arc syndrome
A condition in which raising the arm between the range of 45 and 160 degrees at the side of the body causes pain. The syndrome is caused by inflammation of the tendons or small fluid-filled sacs (bursae) around the shoulder joint. Treatment, if needed, usually includes rest, physical therapy, NSAIDs such as aspirin, and corticosteroid injections.

Periostitis
Painful inflammation of the tissue that covers bone (periosteum), usually caused by injury or infection.

Perthes' disease
Painful inflammation of the head of the thighbone (femur) in children (usually boys), thought to be caused by a disruption in blood supply. Treatment may include bed rest, splinting, or surgery.

Plantar fasciitis
Painful inflammation of connective tissue in the sole of the foot, usually at the point of the heel. Treatment may include use of protective insoles, bed rest, NSAIDs such as aspirin, and corticosteroid injections. Surgery is needed in some cases.

Pseudarthrosis
A false joint in a bone, created either by a disorder such as an unhealed fracture or, rarely, by surgery to restore joint mobility and reduce pain.

Pseudogout
A goutlike joint disorder in which calcium pyrophosphate crystals are deposited in joints. Treatment may include NSAIDs such as aspirin, bed rest, and the injection of a corticosteroid.

Psoriatic arthritis
A form of arthritis that develops in people with psoriasis (a chronic skin disease). The fingernails may be pitted.

R - S

Rheumatology
The branch of medicine concerned with the diagnosis and treatment of diseases of the joints and connective tissues.

Sacroiliitis
Inflammation of the sacroiliac joint in the lower part of the back, caused by arthritis.

Sever's disease
In childhood, painful inflammation of the projecting part of the heel bone (calcaneus). The condition may be caused by chronic strain around the insertion site of the *Achilles tendon*. In most cases, no treatment is needed except padding the shoe.

Spasm
Prolonged, painful, strong contraction of a muscle.

Still's disease
A form of rheumatoid arthritis that affects children.

Subluxation
Partial dislocation of a joint.

Synovial biopsy
A diagnostic procedure in which a sample of the joint lining (synovial membrane) is removed for analysis.

T-V

Tarsal tunnel syndrome
A condition characterized by numbness, tingling, and pain in the foot due to pressure on a nerve as it passes via the ankle into the foot. Surgery may be needed to relieve symptoms.

Temporomandibular joint syndrome
A condition characterized by headache, facial pain, and restriction of jaw movement caused by spasm of the chewing muscles or movement or displacement of the jaw (temporomandibular) joint.

Tendinitis
Inflammation of a tendon, usually caused by injury or by overuse of the tendon. Treatment may include rest, physical therapy, NSAIDs such as aspirin, and, in some cases, corticosteroid injections.

Tophus
Formation of uric acid crystals around joints and the outer ear.

Vertebra
One of the 33 bones of the spinal column.

INDEX

Page numbers in *italics* refer to illustrations and captions. See also the DRUG INDEX on page 139 and the GLOSSARY OF TERMS AND DISORDERS on pages 140 to 141.

Photograph sources:
Biophoto Associates **62** (top right); **62** (top
   center); **90** (center); **110**
The Bridgeman Art Library **9**
Dr Stephen Gwyther **67**; **116**
The Image Bank **7**; **17**; **57**; **95** (bottom left);
   104
Institute of Orthopaedics, UK, **127**
National Medical Slide Bank, UK **61**; **62**
   (bottom center); **90** (bottom left);
   121; **126**
Pictor International **29**; **31**
Saint Bartholomew's Hospital **63** (bottom
   right); **92** (center)
Saint Mary's Hospital **91**; **92** (bottom right);
   98; **101**
Science Photo Library **2** (bottom right); **14**;
   15; **18**; **27**; **46**; **47**; **48**; **49** (bottom right);
   50 (top left); **52**; **54**; **58**; **59** (top left); **62**
   (bottom right); **63** (top right); **70** (top);
   72; **80** (bottom); **90** (bottom right);

95 (center); **100**
The Telegraph Colour Library **30**
Dr Ian Williams **50** (bottom left); **50** (bottom
   right); **51**; **70** (center); **80** (top left); **84**; **93**
   (bottom); **125**
Dr Robert Youngson **70** (bottom)
Zefa Pictures **2** (bottom left); **39**; **81**; **115**

Front cover photograph: Zefa Pictures

**The joint prostheses on page 83
appear courtesy of:**
Smith and Nephew Richards Ltd, UK

**The equipment on pages 88-89
appears courtesy of:**
John Bell and Croyden Ltd, UK

Illustrators:
Karen Cochrane
David Fathers
Tony Graham
Andrew Green
Coral Mula
Gilly Newman
Philip Wilson
John Woodcock

**Commissioned
photography:**
Steve Bartholomew
Yaël Freudmann
Susanna Price
Airbrushing:
Paul Desmond
Roy Flooks
Janos Marffy

Index: Sue Bosanko

Reader's Digest Fund for the Blind is
publisher of the Large-Type Edition of
Reader's Digest. For subscription information about this magazine, please
contact Reader's Digest Fund for the
Blind, Inc., Dept. 250, Pleasantville, N.Y.
10570.